Open, Laparoscopic and Robotic Hepatic Transection

Isidoro Di Carlo
Editor

Open, Laparoscopic and Robotic Hepatic Transection

Tools and Methods

Foreword by Jacques Belghiti

Springer

Editor
Isidoro Di Carlo
Department of Surgical Sciences
Organ Transplantation and Advanced Technologies
Cannizzaro Hospital
University of Catania
Catania
Italy

Additional material to this book can be downloaded from http://extras.springer.com/

ISBN 978-88-470-2621-6 ISBN 978-88-470-2622-3 (eBook)
DOI 10.1007/978-88-470-2622-3
Springer Milan Heidelberg New York Dordrecht London

Library of Congress Control Number: 2012944389

Printed on acid-free paper

Springer is part of Springer Science+Business Media (www.springer.com)

To my wife and my sons

Foreword

I read this last book by Professor Isidoro Di Carlo, which explicitly focuses on the most challenging step of liver resection, parenchymal transection, with great interest. The laparoscopic approach is now challenging laparotomy and will gain the upper hand in the future. Liver surgery requires an extensive knowledge of the segmental and subsegmental liver anatomy. This perception is facilitated by 3D preoperative reconstruction, which will be enriched by intraoperative navigation. After more or less extensive mobilization of the liver, the parenchymal transection has multiple and parallel goals. The first objective is to leave a well-vascularized remnant liver with adequate outflow in order to optimize hepatic function and to ensure good regeneration. This often requires the preservation of the hepatic veins with a good flow. The second goal is to ensure both good hemostasis and biliostasis. Hemostasis, which was the priority of liver surgeons many years ago, is now efficiently achieved by all the procedures described in this book. In contrast, biliostasis remains a problem and liver surgeons are still concerned with the undiminished rate of postoperative biliary fistula, which prolongs the hospital stay. Regardless of the quality of biliostasis, the risk of biliary leak increases when liver resection exposes the biliary confluence or after resection of segment 8. Since the vast majority of liver resections are indicated for malignant tumors, the last concern is the choice of the best oncologic plane. It is now well established that anatomic resection is the best extent of resection for HCC. For many years, Makuuchi has shown that resection of the tumor in combination with its vascular territory decreases the risk of local recurrence. The oncologic plane of liver metastasis is different with a margin width taking into account the persistence of peripheral malignant cells after several cycles of chemotherapy. The oncologic plane of biliary tumors, which can spread along the biliary tract and are often associated with satellite nodules, remains to be defined.

All transection procedures described in this manual by top world surgeons pursue these goals. I'm confident that all surgeons will find valuable methods among the broad variety presented.

Jacques Belghiti, MD

Preface

The hepatic surgery developed slowly until the middle of the nineteenth century, when the knowledge of the anatomy permitted a radical change in the feasibility of the surgical approach to the liver diseases. The perfect understanding of the hepatic segmental structures allowed to perform all kind of the hepatic resection. In the last two decades the refinements of diagnostic methods, and anesthetic improvements have allowed to achieve more satisfactory results. The most important cause of post-operative morbidity and mortality, is still related to the transection of the liver that represents the key moment in the hepatic surgery.

Before the advent of laparoscopic and robotic surgery the hepatic transection was almost ever performed through the kelly clasia method. Although many methods were available, the Kelly was reputed the mandatory tool to achieve liver transection for a long time.

With the advent of laparoscopy first and robotic thereafter, this solid statement changed. With these revolutionary methods several tools became mandatory to achieve hepatic transection.

The aim of this textbook is to describe all the tools that can actually be used to perform hepatic resection in open, laparoscopic, and robotic surgery. To achieve this at the best, I asked to the most reputed hepatic surgeons in the world to describe their techniques with the tools they have patented or simply used. My grateful thanks to all the surgeons listed in this book.

Isidoro Di Carlo

Preface

Contents

Contributors

Luca Aldrighetti Hepatobiliary Surgery Unit, Department of Surgery, San Raffaele Hospital, Vita-Salute San Raffaele University, Milan, Italy

Keith M. Baldwin Department of Surgery, Roger Williams Medical Center, Providence, RI, USA

Andrea Belli Department of General and Hepato-Pancreato-Biliary Surgery, S.M. Loreto Nuovo Hospital, Naples, Italy

Giulio Belli Department of General and Hepato-Pancreato-Biliary Surgery, S.M. Loreto Nuovo Hospital, Naples, Italy

Helge Bruns Department of General and Transplant Surgery, Ruprecht-Karls-University, Heidelberg, Germany

Markus W. Büchler Department of General and Transplant Surgery, Ruprecht-Karls-University, Heidelberg, Germany

Xiu Jun Cai Department of Surgery, Sir Run Run Shaw Hospital, Zhejiang University, Hangzhou, Zhejiang, People's Republic of China

Isidoro Di Carlo Department of Surgical Sciences, Organ Transplantation and Advanced Technologies, Cannizzaro Hospital, University of Catania, Catania, Italy

Marco Catena Department of Surgery, Hepatobiliary Surgery Unit, San Raffaele Hospital, Vita-Salute San Raffaele University, Milan, Italy

Yu-Chung Chang Department of Surgery, Medical College and Hospital, National Cheng Kung University, Tainan, Taiwan, Republic of China

Deepak Chhabra Department of Surgical Oncology, Lilavati Hospital and Research Centre, Mumbai, India

Gi-Hong Choi Department of Surgery, Yonsei University Health System, Seoul, Republic of Korea

Luigi Cioffi Department of General and Hepato-Pancreato-Biliary Surgery, S.M. Loreto Nuovo Hospital, Naples, Italy

Federica Cipriani Hepatobiliary Surgery Unit, Department of Surgery, San Raffaele Hospital, Vita-Salute San Raffaele University, Milan, Italy

Alberto D'Agostino Department of General and Hepato-Pancreato-Biliary Surgery, S.M. Loreto Nuovo Hospital, Naples, Italy

Matteo Donadon Liver Surgery Unit, Department of General Surgery, IRCCS Istituto Clinico Humanitas, University of Milan, Milan, Italy

Denis Ehrl Surgical Department of Visceral and Thoracic Surgery, Amper Klinikum Dachau, Dachau, Germany

Giorgio Ercolani Department of Surgery and Transplantation, Sant'Orsola Hospital, University of Bologna, Bologna, Italy

Corrado Fantini Department of General and Hepato-Pancreato-Biliary Surgery, S.M. Loreto Nuovo Hospital, Naples, Italy

Brice Gayet Département de Pathologie Digestive, L'Institut Mutualiste Monsouris, Paris, France

Paolo Di Gioia Department of Surgery and Transplantation, Sant'Orsola Hospital, University of Bologna, Bologna, Italy

Nagy A. Habib HPB Surgery, Hammersmith Hospital, Imperial College London, London, UK

Takuya Hashimoto Department of Hepato-Biliary-Pancreatic Surgery, Japanese Red Cross Medical Center, University of Tokyo, Shibuya-ku, Tokyo, Japan

Kerstin Huepgens Surgical Department of Visceral and Thoracic Surgery, Amper Klinikum Dachau, Dachau, Germany

Palepu Jagannath Department of Surgical Oncology, Lilavati Hospital and Research Centre, Mumbai, India

N. Joseph Espat Department of Surgery, Roger Williams Medical Center, Providence, RI, USA

Hironori Kaneko Faculty of Medicine, Department of Surgery (Omori), Toho University, Otaku, Tokyo, Japan

Ki-Hun Kim Division of Hepatobiliary Surgery and Liver Transplantation, Department of Surgery, Asan Medical Center, Ulsan University, Seoul, Republic of Korea

Steven C. Katz Department of Surgery, Roger Williams Medical Center, Providence, RI, USA

Hiroaki Kitade Surgery, Kansai Medical University, Hirakata, Osaka, Japan

Norihiro Kokudo Department of Hepato-Biliary-Pancreatic Surgery, Department of Artificial Organ and Transplantation, Graduate School of Medicine, University of Tokyo, Bunkyo-ku, Tokyo, Japan

Michael Kremer Department of General and Transplant Surgery, Ruprecht-Karls-University, Heidelberg, Germany

A-Hon Kwon Surgery Kansai Medical University, Hirakata, Osaka, Japan

Charis Kyriakides HPB Surgery, Hammersmith Hospital, Imperial College London, London, UK

Jiang Tao Li Department of Surgery, Second Affiliated Hospital, Zhejiang University Medical School, Hangzhou, Zhejiang, People's Republic of China

Paolo Limongelli Department of General and Hepato-Pancreato-Biliary Surgery, S.M. Loreto Nuovo Hospital, Naples, Italy

Masatoshi Makuuchi Department of Hepato-Biliary-Pancreatic Surgery, Japanese Red Cross Medical Center, University of Tokyo, Shibuya-ku, Tokyo, Japan

Yoichi Matsui Surgery, Kansai Medical University, Hirakata, Osaka, Japan

Yuichiro Otsuka Faculty of Medicine, Department of Surgery (Omori), Toho University, Otaku, Tokyo, Japan

Michele Paganelli Hepatobiliary Surgery Unit, Department of Surgery, San Raffaele Hospital, Vita-Salute San Raffaele University, Milan, Italy

Madhava Pai HPB Surgery, Hammersmith Hospital, Imperial College London, London, UK

Shu You Peng Department of Surgery, Second Affiliated Hospital and Sir Run Run Shaw Hospital, Zhejiang University Medical School, Hangzhou, Zhejiang, People's Republic of China

Antonio Daniele Pinna Department of Surgery and Transplantation, Sant'Orsola Hospital, University of Bologna, Bologna, Italy

Francesca Ratti Hepatobiliary Surgery Unit, Department of Surgery, San Raffaele Hospital, Vita-Salute San Raffaele University, Milan, Italy

Horst-Guenter Rau Surgical Department of Visceral and Thoracic Surgery, Amper Klinikum Dachau, Dachau, Germany?

Matteo Ravaioli Department of Surgery and Transplantation, Sant'Orsola Hospital, University of Bologna, Bologna, Italy

Gianluca Russo Department of General and Hepato-Pancreato-Biliary Surgery, S.M. Loreto Nuovo Hospital, Naples, Italy

Akio Saiura Department of Gastroenterological Surgery, Cancer Institute Ariake Hospital, Japanese Foundation for Cancer Research, Tokyo, Japan

Sohei Satoi Surgery, Kansai Medical University, Hirakata, Osaka, Japan

Peter Schemmer Department of General and Transplant Surgery, Ruprecht-Karls-University, Heidelberg, Germany

Matteo Serenari Department of Surgery and Transplantation, Sant'Orsola Hospital, University of Bologna, Bologna, Italy

Rajiv Shah Department of Surgical Oncology, Lilavati Hospital and Research Centre, Mumbai, India

Ponnandai Somasundar Department of Surgery, Roger Williams Medical Center, Providence, RI, USA

Zhi Jian Tan Department of Surgery, Second Affiliated Hospital, Guangzhou University of Chinese Medicine, Guangzhou, Guangdong, People's Republic of China

Adriana Toro Department of Surgical Sciences, Organ Transplantation and Advanced Technologies, Cannizzaro Hospital, University of Catania, Catania, Italy

Guido Torzilli Liver Surgery Unit, Department of General Surgery, IRCCS Istituto Clinico Humanitas, University of Milan, Milan, Italy

Yi Fan Wang Department of Surgery, Sir Run Run Shaw Hospital, Zhejiang University, Hangzhou, Zhejiang, People's Republic of China

Jürgen Weitz Department of General and Transplant Surgery, Ruprecht-Karls-University, Heidelberg, Germany

Feng Xi HPB Surgery, Hammersmith Hospital, Imperial College London, London, UK

Junji Yamamoto Department of Surgery, National Defense Medical College, Saitama, Japan

Noah B. Zuker Département de Pathologie Digestive, L'Institut Mutualiste Monsouris, Paris, France

Part I
Open Hepatic Transection

Open Hepatic Transection Using Microwave Tissue Coagulation

1

Sohei Satoi, Hiroaki Kitade, Yoichi Matsui and A-Hon Kwon

1.1 Introduction

As a result of improvements in the safety of hepatic parenchymal resection within the past few decades, liver resection has become a widely accepted treatment modality for various benign and malignant hepatobiliary diseases [1]. As post-operative mortality and morbidity rates have decreased, the number of liver resections performed to treat liver tumors has increased. The primary factors underlying these improvements include methods used to limit intraoperative blood loss (e.g., advances in hepatic imaging and surgical technique), enhanced understanding of hepatic anatomy, and perioperative management [1]. To achieve safe and effective liver transection, various surgical techniques have been introduced and used in clinical practice; For example, to reduce intraoperative blood loss, which can lead to postoperative complications and shorten survival time, surgeons use Pringle's maneuver [2], hypotensive anesthetics [3], infrahepatic inferior vena cava clamping [4], and various devices for transecting the liver parenchyma [4–6].

Microwave tissue coagulation (MTC) was developed in 1979 by Tabuse et al. [7] and has been applied clinically for transection of hepatic parenchyma with or without liver cirrhosis. Use of MTC has been reported to reduce blood loss and to

Electronic Supplementary Material The online version of this article (doi:10.1007/978-88-470-2622-3_1) contains supplementary material which is available to authorized users.

S. Satoi (✉)
Surgery, Kansai Medical University,
Hirakata, Osaka, Japan
e-mail: satoi@hirakata.kmu.ac.jp

I. Di Carlo (ed.), *Open, Laparoscopic and Robotic Hepatic Transection*,
DOI: 10.1007/978-88-470-2622-3_1, © Springer-Verlag Italia 2012

enable nonanatomical liver resections, even in patients with poor liver functional reserve [7–10].

In Asia, most patients with hepatocellular carcinoma (HCC) have underlying viral hepatitis, and the extent of liver resection can be limited by poor liver functional reserve. Nonanatomical liver resection is sometimes necessary in this situation, and it is important to control intraoperative blood loss. Therefore, between 1992 and 2005, we routinely used MTC to minimize the amount of liver resection needed based on tumor size. This type of hepatic transection is easy to perform and does not require special surgical techniques.

Our standard procedure for surgical treatment of HCC has been to minimize the extent of liver resection and to avoid performing Pringle's maneuver because of the risk of ischemic injury to the liver. Hence, we used MTC to perform nonanatomical liver resections, taking into account tumor size. We previously reported that, in 214 patients with HCC who underwent nonanatomical liver resections between 1992 and 2001, MTC was used safely with no need for special surgical techniques, and acceptable long-term results were achieved [9, 10]. Moreover, we have recommended no-margin resection using MTC in HCC patients with limited liver functional reserve and with tumors that are centrally located and close to large hepatic vascular structures [11].

In this chapter, we describe the MTC device, surgical indications, and surgical technique, illustrated with photographs and video on the use of MTC for open hepatic transection.

1.2 Device Description

Microwave Tissue Coagulator. Basic information about the MTC and its clinical applications have been reported in detail by Tabuse, who was a pioneer in the surgical application of microwave radiation [12]. The heating method used to coagulate tissue is mainly classified as external heating or internal heating. External heating coagulates tissue by conducting heat from the surface to the inside of tissue (e.g., laser and heat probe methods). For internal heating, an MTC device is used to coagulate tissue by internal heating via a coaxial needle antenna. The microwave radiation is absorbed well due to water molecule resonance in tissue with high fluid volume (e.g., muscle, parenchymal organs, and blood). The microwave heating process is affected not only by free water molecules in the tissue but also by water molecules bound to the structure of large biomolecules. Heat is produced by the vibrational energy of polar substances in protein and water molecules, as well as when water undergoes dissociation, and polarity is lost due to protein coagulation. Heating after completion of coagulation will cause dissociation of water, resulting in no further heat generation. Therefore, microwave coagulation fields do not propagate in tissue as plane waves, so energy absorption is limited to tissue near the coaxial needle antenna.

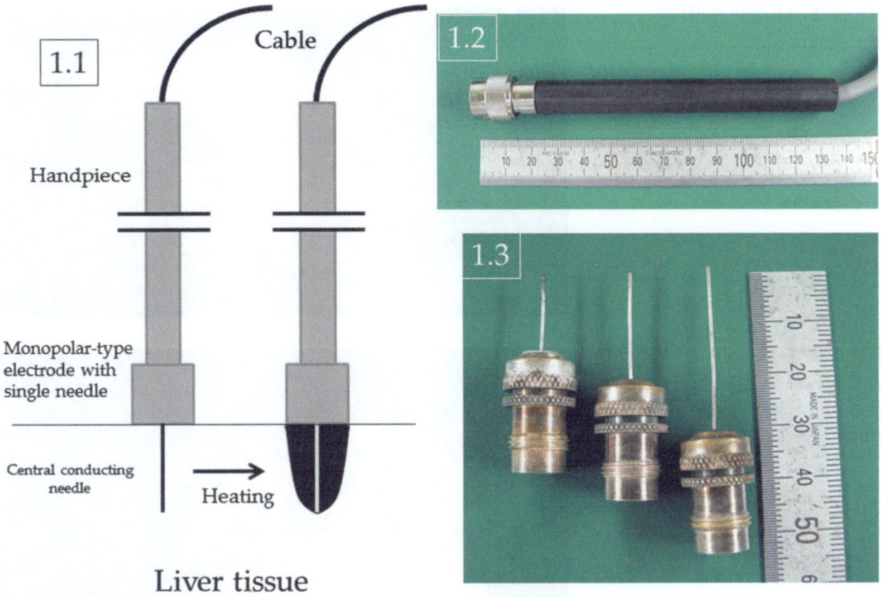

Fig. 1.1 **a** Coagulation area produced by the MTC electrode. The *black area* surrounding the needle electrode represents the coagulation area. **b** Handpiece of MTC device. **c** Needle applicator consisting of a 15-, 20-, or 30-mm-long electrode and its base

Figure 1.1 shows the coagulation area produced by a surgical electrode; the size of the area depends on the length of the antenna. The MTC device consists of a basic needle applicator and a 2.45-GHz (150 W) generator (Microtaze^{TM}; Alfresa Co., Osaka, Japan). This microwave system can burn tissue and ablate all tissue structures, including major blood vessels, within the microwave field; For example, the MTC device heats liver parenchyma to produce coagulation by internal radiation via the coaxial needle antenna. For liver resection, monopolar-type electrodes with single or double needles are available. We have used the single-needle electrode for transection of hepatic parenchyma. As shown in Figs. 1.2 and 1.3, the needle applicator consists of an electrode (with length of 15, 20 or 30 mm) and its base, which is attached to the handpiece. To insert the needle electrode into the hepatic parenchyma at the subphrenic space (the narrow space between the liver and the diaphragm), an L-shaped connector can be placed between the base of the needle electrode and the handpiece. In our experience, the range of power applied was 60–80 W, and coagulation and dissociation times were 45 and 15 s, respectively. The power selected was 60 W for noncirrhotic liver and 80 W for cirrhotic liver. Coagulated liver tissue often adheres tightly to the tip of the electrode during heating, which makes it difficult to separate the electrode from the tissue after completing coagulation. If the electrode is pulled out using any force, the coagulated tissue may bleed. To avoid this problem, a dissociation device delivers negative voltage to the central conductor of the electrode and positive voltage to the

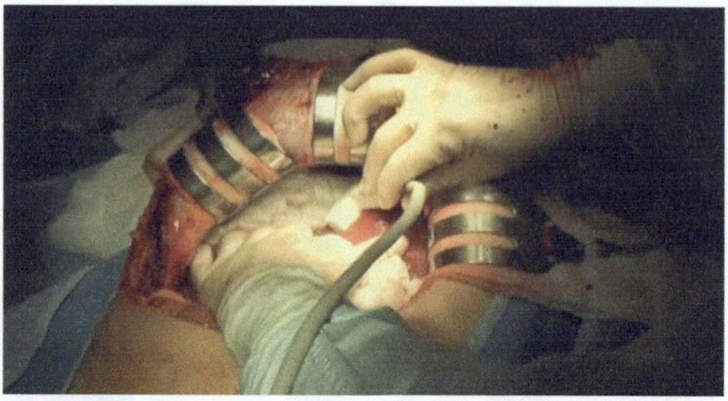

Fig. 1.2 Intraoperative ultrasonography

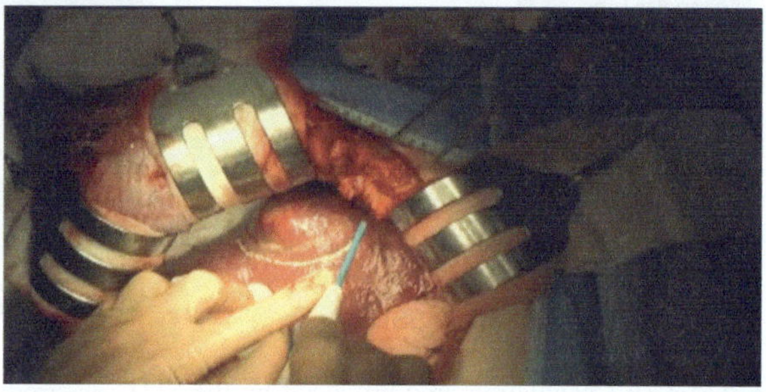

Fig. 1.3 Intended transection line 1 cm away from the tumor along the tumor's circumference

electrode's outer conductor. As a result, electro-osmosis causes water to gather around the central conductor of the electrode, which softens the dry tissue adhered to the electrode. Consequently, the electrode can be easily separated from the liver tissue.

1.3 Technique Description, Complications, and Results

1.3.1 Surgical Indication for Microwave Surgery

Both surgical efficacy and postoperative liver functional reserve are generally considered crucial for successful treatment of patients with HCC. In Japan, anatomical liver resection is preferred over nonanatomical resection for eradicating intrahepatic metastases confined to tumor-bearing portal tributaries. There have been no randomized clinical trials investigating survival based on the extent of liver resection. However, in several case series, nonanatomical liver resection has been shown to produce survival results similar to those associated with anatomical resection [11, 13, 14], while other studies have demonstrated the survival benefits of anatomical liver resection for HCC patients [15, 16]. Nonanatomical liver resection performed using MTC is useful for: (1) HCC patients with poor liver functional reserve (which is a contraindication to anatomical liver resection), (2) patients with HCC located at a border between different liver segments, and (3) patients with metastatic liver tumors that are not associated with intrahepatic metastases confined to tumor-bearing portal tributaries.

1.3.2 MTC Technique Description

After laparotomy, the tumor location and its relationship to the Glissonian sheaths or hepatic veins are determined using intraoperative ultrasonography. The hepatic parenchyma is coagulated during repeated insertions of a monopolar-type single-needle electrode along the intended resection line, 1–3 cm away from the tumor, depending on the tumor's diameter. After coagulation is performed using the needle electrode, the liver's surface changes color over an area approximately 1 cm in diameter around the base of the needle electrode. The first session of MTC ablation of hepatic parenchyma using MTC can be performed under the guidance of ultrasonography. Before the first session, the depth and direction of needle electrode insertion should be designed to create a cone-shaped coagulation area that extends beneath the tumor, because the presence of coagulated parenchyma can interfere with ultrasonographic examination after several sessions. The needle electrode is inserted into the liver tissue every 1 cm along the circumferential resection line, with care taken to avoid puncturing the Glissonian sheaths and hepatic veins. The hepatic parenchyma is transected through the center of the ablation zone using the clamp-crushing method with forceps but without Pringle's maneuver. Any visible exposed blood vessels and the Glissonian sheaths are ligated with sutures to avoid postoperative bleeding and bile leakage.

When liver resection with hepaticojejunostomy is planned, use of MTC should be avoided. It is possible that intestinal bacteria could easily reach the coagulated stump of the hepatic parenchyma after hepaticojejunostomy, resulting in abscess formation.

1.3.3 A Case Presentation

A 60-year-old man (height, 174 cm; weight, 85.4 kg; body mass index, 28.2 kg/m^2) who had type B hepatitis was clinically diagnosed with HCC. Abdominal contrast-enhanced computed tomography scanning showed a mass approximately 50 mm in diameter on liver segment VIII. The patient's blood cell count and biochemical test results were as follows: prothrombin time, 101 %; white blood cells, 5,000/μl; hemoglobin, 14.5 g/dl; platelet count, 13.1×10^4/μl; fasting blood sugar, 107 mg/dl; serum albumin, 4.0 g/dl; alpha-fetoprotein, 18.3 ng/dl; and L3 fraction, 21.1 %. Technetium-99m-galactosyl human serum albumin liver scintigraphy showed a total Rmax value of 0.603 mg/min, indicating the presence of chronic hepatitis or mild liver cirrhosis, and the indocyanine green retention rate at 15 min (ICG-R15) was 13.4 % (normal range, 0–10 %). The patient was scheduled to undergo nonanatomical liver resection using MTC.

Upon open laparotomy, there were no signs of ascites, peritoneal seeding, or other organ metastases. After mobilization of the liver, intraoperative ultrasonography showed the presence of the tumor 50 mm in diameter on segment VIII, with no satellite lesions of HCC in the liver. Moreover, the position of the tumor

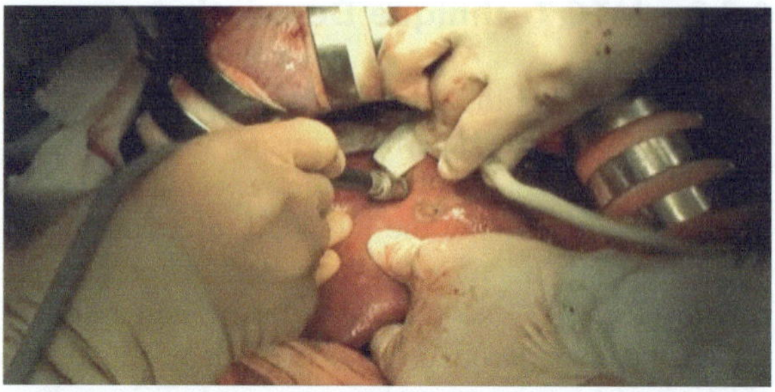

Fig. 1.4 First session of MTC ablation of hepatic parenchyma performed under guidance of ultrasonography

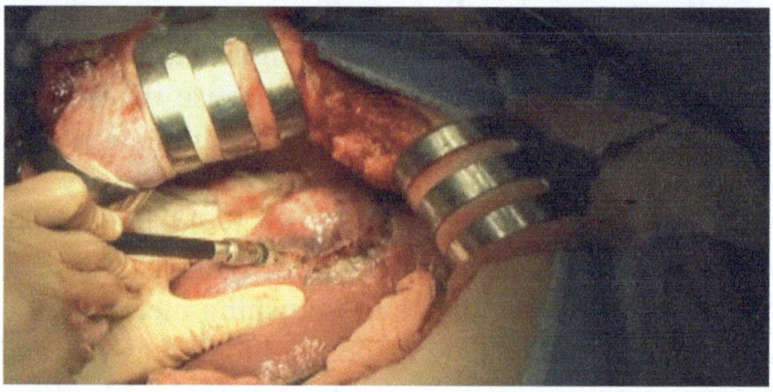

Fig. 1.5 Surface of liver tissue after several sessions of MTC

relative to the major blood vessels and the Glissonian sheaths was confirmed using intraoperative ultrasonography, in order to avoid MTC damage of the latter structures (Fig. 1.2). The direction and depth of the coagulation puncture line were then decided based on the liver volume to be resected and the positions of the major blood vessels and Glissonian sheaths. The intended transection line was delineated, keeping it 1 cm away from the tumor along the tumor's circumference (Fig. 1.3). The MTC needle electrode was inserted to create cone-shaped coagulation areas at 1-cm intervals along the transection line. The first session of MTC ablation of hepatic parenchyma was performed under the guidance of ultrasonography (Fig. 1.4). The surface of the liver tissue changed color and contracted after completion of several sessions of MTC (Fig. 1.5). Because the tumor was located at a subphrenic space, it was impossible to puncture the dorsal side of the tumor with the long, straight type of needle applicator. In this situation, the L-shaped connector between the base of the needle electrode and the handpiece was used to allow easy insertion (Fig. 1.6). Special attention should be paid to prevent injury of the Glissonian sheaths and hepatic veins, thus avoiding post-operative bile leakage or venous bleeding. After repeated MTC ablation along the intended transection line, the coagulated hepatic parenchyma was transected using the clamp-crushing method with forceps but without performing Pringle's maneuver (Fig. 1.7). Visible exposed blood vessels and Glissonian sheaths were carefully ligated and cut (Fig. 1.8). Finally, the Glissonian sheath of segment VIII was exposed and ligated with stitches, and liver resection was completed (Fig. 1.9). After peritoneal lavage using natural saline (3,000 ml) and confirmation of hemostasis, a closed-suction drain was inserted. The abdominal wall was closed

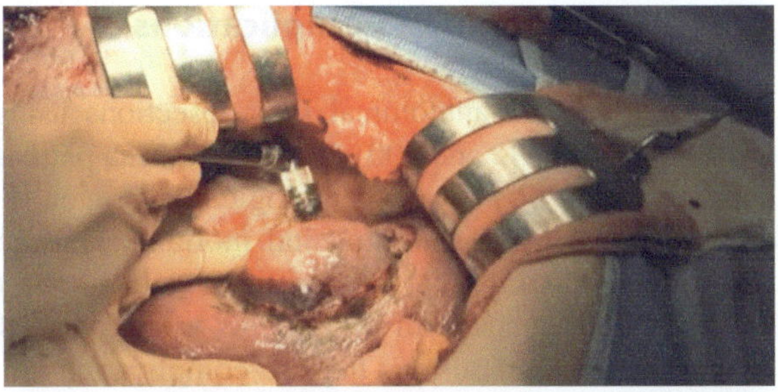

Fig. 1.6 Use of L-shaped connector at the dorsal side of the tumor

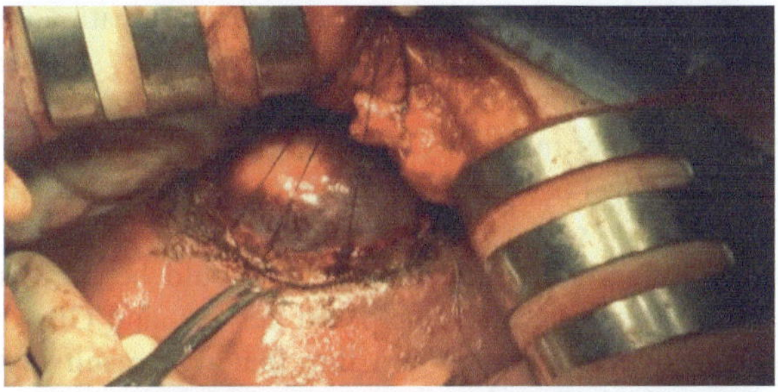

Fig. 1.7 Hepatic transection using the clamp-crushing method with forceps but without Pringle's maneuver

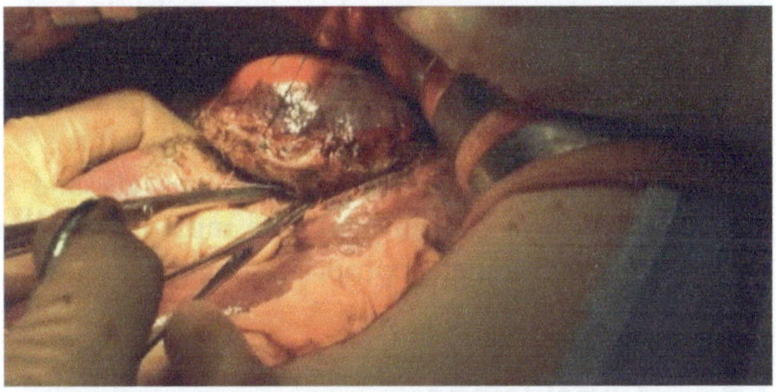

Fig. 1.8 Ligation and cutting of the exposed blood vessels and Glissonian sheaths

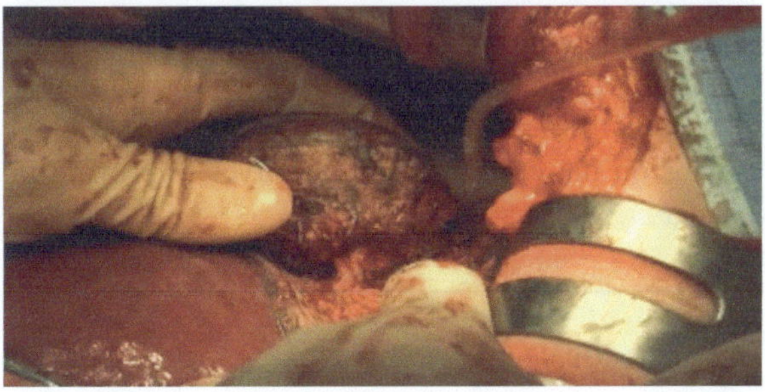

Fig. 1.9 Exposure of the Glissonian sheath of liver segment VIII

in three layers. The operative time was 4 h 47 min, and the volume of blood loss was 60 ml. The postoperative course was uneventful, and the patient was discharged on postoperative day 14. Pathological examination showed moderately differentiated HCC with clear surgical margins.

1.3.4 Postoperative Complications

We performed nonanatomical liver resections using MTC in 214 patients with HCC between 1992 and 2001 [9, 10]. Of these patients, 72 % suffered from type C hepatitis and 47 % had pathologically proven liver cirrhosis. Postoperative morbidity was 36 %, and hospital mortality was 2.8 %. Intractable bile leakage was observed in 1.4 % of these patients, and 13 % exhibited abscess formation on the liver's cut surface. In 99 patients treated for HCC between 1984 and 1999, Ryu et al. reported serious hepatic complications in 13.1 %, including 9 % with bile leakage, and the hospital mortality rate was 3 % [8].

In a comparison of postoperative complications in patients with high (>20 %) versus low ($\leq$20 %) ICG-R15 values, no significant difference in morbidity between the low- and high-ICG-R15 groups was found, but there was a trend toward higher morbidity in the high-ICG-R15 group (morbidity rate, 41 % versus 29 %) [10]. Postoperative complications in most patients were well controlled.

Guidelines to Prevent Pitfalls:

1. Before MTC, ultrasonography should be used: (a) to determine the relative positions of the tumor, blood vessels, and Glissonian sheaths, and (b) to plan the intended transection line that will result in the *cone-shaped coagulation area* including the tumor.
2. To prevent postoperative bleeding and bile leakage, it is critical: (a) to avoid coagulating the major blood vessels and Glissonian sheaths via inadvertent contact with the MTC needle electrode, and (b) to carefully ligate and cut the visible blood vessels and Glissonian sheaths.
3. To easily detect the small blood vessels and Glissonian sheaths: (a) good visualization of the surgical area must be maintained, and (b) dissection must be performed under appropriate countertraction.

1.4 Conclusions

Hepatic transection performed using MTC, while taking into account the tumor size, is a safe procedure and does not require other special surgical techniques. It is important to carefully ligate and cut the visible blood vessels and Glissonian sheaths on the cut surface of the liver to prevent postoperative bleeding and bile leakage.

References

1. Jarnagin WR, Gonen M, Fong Y et al. (2002) Improvement in perioperative outcome after hepatic resection: analysis of 1,803 consecutive cases over the past decade. Ann Surg 236:397–406
2. Pringle JH (1908) Notes on the arrest of hepatic hemorrhage due to trauma. Ann Surg 48:541–549

3. Rahbari NN, Koch M, Zimmermann JB, Elbers H et al. (2011) Infrahepatic inferior vena cava clamping for reduction of central venous pressure and blood loss during hepatic resection: a randomized controlled trial. Ann Surg 253:1102–1110
4. Takayama T, Makuuchi M, Kubota K et al. (2001) Randomized comparison of ultrasonic vs clamp transection of the liver. Arch Surg 136:922–928
5. Papachristou DN, Barters R (1982) Resection of the liver with a water jet. Br J Surg 69:93–94
6. Schmidbauer S, Hallfeldt KK, Sitzmann G et al. (2002) Experience with ultrasound scissors and blades (UltraCision) in open and laparoscopic liver resection. Ann Surg 235:27–30
7. Tabuse K, Katsumi M, Kobayashi Y et al. (1985) Microwave surgery: hepatectomy using a microwave tissue coagulator. World J Surg 9:136–143
8. Ryu M, Watanabe K, Yamamoto H (1998) Hepatectomy with microwave tissue coagulation for hepatocellular carcinoma. J Hep Bil Pancr Surg 5:184–191
9. Satoi S, Kamiyama Y, Matsui Y et al. (2005) Clinical outcome of 214 liver resections using microwave tissue coagulation. Hepatogastroenterology 52:1180–1185
10. Satoi S, Matsui Y, Kitade H et al. (2008) Long-term outcome of hepatocellular carcinoma patients who underwent liver resection using microwave tissue coagulation. HPB 10:289–295
11. Matsui Y, Terakawa N, Satoi S et al. (2007) Postoperative outcomes in patients with hepatocellular carcinomas resected with exposure of the tumor surface clinical role of the no-margin resection. Arch Surg 142:596–602
12. Tabuse K (1998) Basic knowledge of a microwave tissue coagulator and its clinical applications. J Hepatobiliary Pancreat Surg 5:165–172
13. Eguchi S, Kanematsu T, Arii S et al. (2008) Comparison of the outcomes between an anatomical subsegmentectomy and a non-anatomical minor hepatectomy for single hepatocellular carcinomas based on a Japanese nationwide survey. Surgery 143:469–475
14. Kanematsu T, Takenaka K, Matsumata T et al. (1984) Limited hepatic resection effective for selected cirrhotic patients with primary liver cancer. Ann Surg 199:51–56
15. Regimbeau JM, Kianmanesh R, Farges O et al. (2002) Extent of liver resection influences the outcome in patients with cirrhosis and small hepatocellular carcinoma. Surgery 131:311–317
16. Hasegawa K, Kokudo N, Imamura H et al. (2005) Prognostic impact of anatomic resection for hepatocellular carcinoma. Ann Surg 242(2):252–259

[illegible]

Open Hepatic Transection Using Chang's Needle

2

Yu-Chung Chang

2.1 Introduction

The techniques of hemostasis, inflow and outflow control, and reducing ischemia–reperfusion injuries and tumor cell floating during liver parenchymal transection are the major issues of hepatic resection for benign and malignant liver diseases. Although surgical techniques, sophisticated instruments, and postoperative care are improving, simple, inexpensive, less insult-inducing, less technique- and training-demanding instruments and maneuvers are fundamental for global use. In 1911, a German surgeon, Professor Walther Wendel [1], published a paper about such a preliminary technique. Coincidently, about 100 years later (1996) in Asia, a Taiwanese surgeon [2–4] began innovative techniques by using a similar instrument without knowing about the existence of this pioneer.

2.2 Device Description

Chang's needle consists of a straight, inner needle with a hook near its top to catch the thread, and an 18-gauge stainless-steel external sheath (Fig. 2.1a) to prevent tissue and vascular injuries caused by the hook during the procedure.

Electronic Supplementary Material The online version of this article (doi:10.1007/978-88-470-2622-3_2) contains supplementary material which is available to authorized users.

Y.-C. Chang (✉)
Department of Surgery, Medical College and Hospital, National Cheng Kung University, 138 Sheng-Li Road, Tainan, 70428 Taiwan, Republic of China
e-mail: changmdphd@yahoo.com

I. Di Carlo (ed.), *Open, Laparoscopic and Robotic Hepatic Transection,*
DOI: 10.1007/978-88-470-2622-3_2, © Springer-Verlag Italia 2012

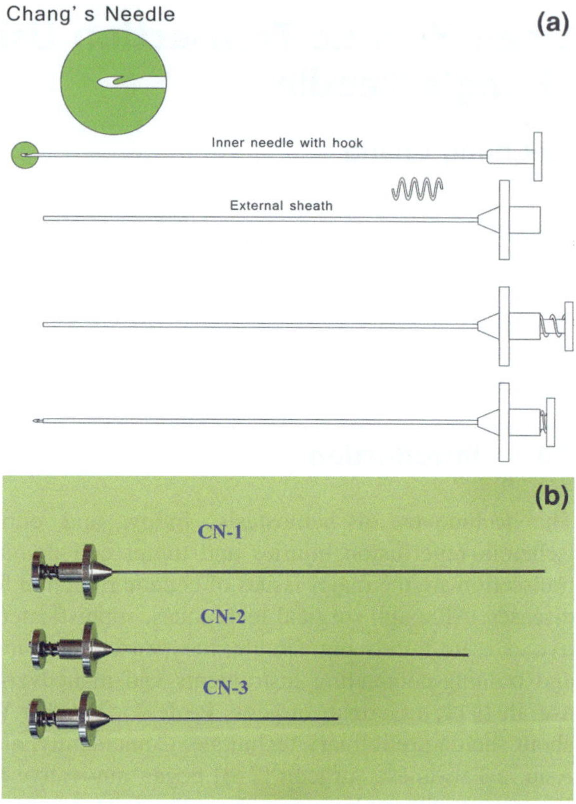

Fig. 2.1 Scheme (**a**) and photos (**b**) of Chang's needle

Currently, we have inner needles of three sizes (19.5, 16.5, and 11.5 cm) to be used for livers of varying sizes and thicknesses (Fig. 2.1b). A curved needle is being developed as well in an effort to control every individual intrahepatic vessel in laparotomy and laparoscopy models.

2.3 Technique Description: Right Hepatic Lobectomy

A right or bilateral subcostal incision with or without extension to the xyphoid is used to open the abdomen. The right side of the liver is first thoroughly mobilized and routinely examined by palpation, and intraoperative ultrasonography is used to confirm the lesion and to determine a suitable division line. Doppler ultrasonography can be used to locate the inflow and outflow vessels if needed. Next, Chang's needle is applied repeatedly along both sides of the division line. The needle penetrates the entire depth of the liver parenchyma from the liver surface and catches one end of no. 1 silk thread from below (Figs. 2.2 and 2.3), then penetrates again, 3–5 cm away from the previous point of insertion, to catch the

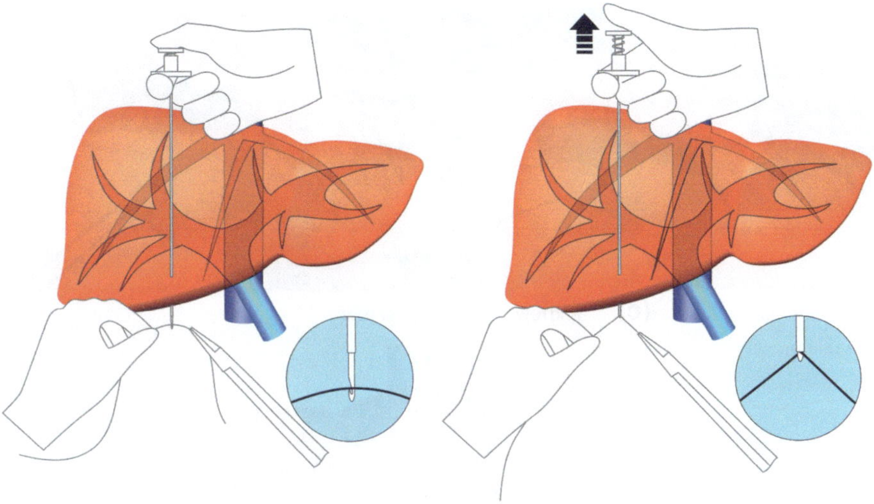

Fig. 2.2 Chang's maneuver for entire-thickness liver puncture

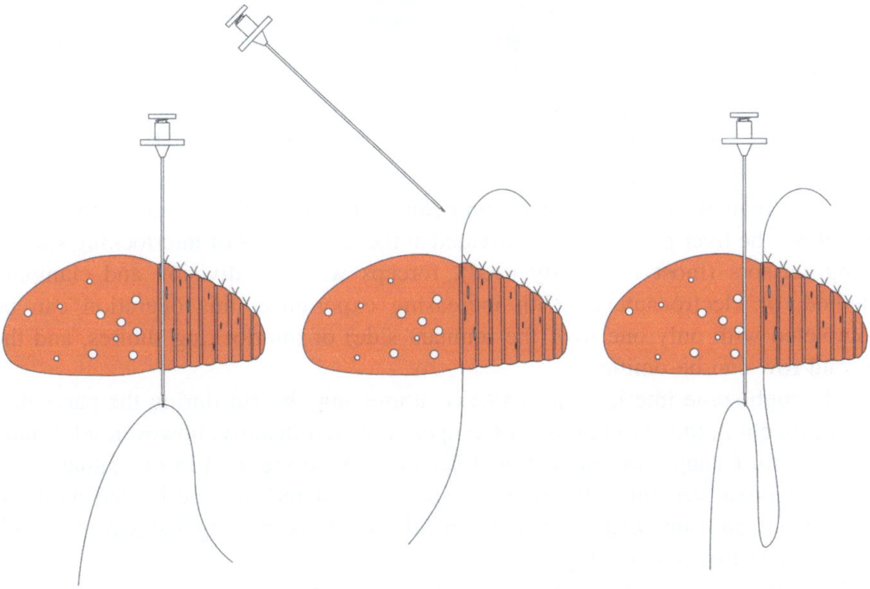

Fig. 2.3 Cross-section view of the interlocking mattress sutures

other end of the thread. A secure tie can subsequently be made to block all vascular flows within this area (Fig. 2.3).

Ultimately, two rows of interlocking mattress sutures are formed (Fig. 2.4a–c). Doppler ultrasonography may alternatively be used to verify whether the vessels are securely blocked before the hepatic transection. Subsequently, without using

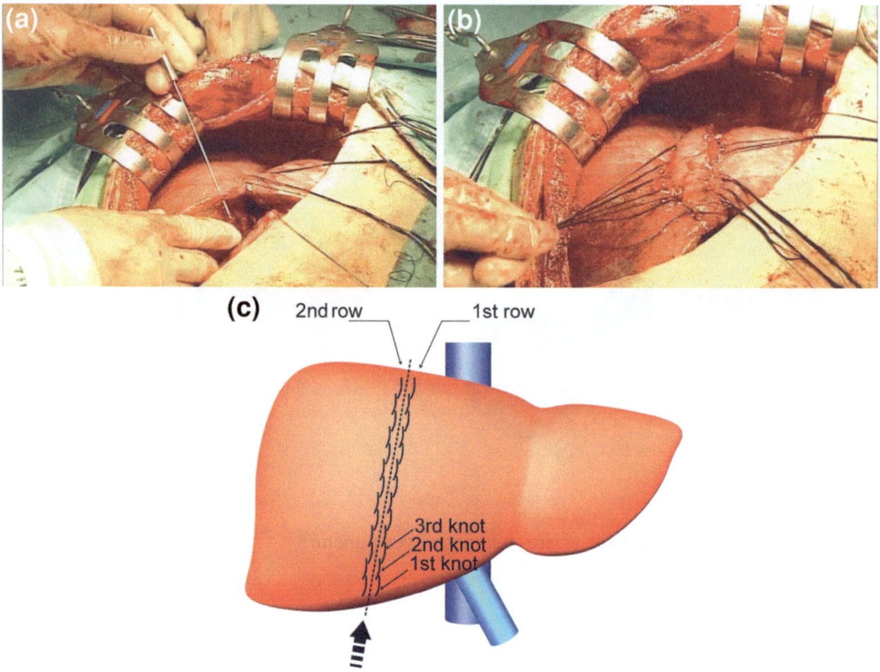

Fig. 2.4 Interlocking mattress sutures or right hepatic lobectomy: **a** finishing the first row and starting the second row puncture; **b**, **c** completion of two rows, but now only one row is necessary

Pringle's maneuver or any other procedures to block the hepatic inflow and backflow, the liver parenchyma is divided at these two rows of interlocking sutures using scissors (most frequently used), forceps with the division and clamping method, or electrocautery. With increasing experience, this operation can be completed with only one row (the remnant side) of interlocking sutures, and the second row can be omitted.

Although some interlocking mattress sutures may be cut during the parenchymal transection, this will not affect the operation significantly; however, additional sutures with Chang's or conventional needle may be required in this situation.

Any tubular structure of significant size encountered may be ligated with 3-0 silk thread, and any major Glission sheath can be suture-ligated with 2-0 silk thread for reinforcement (Fig. 2.5).

Sometimes a congestive condition of the liver may occur and cause unnecessary bleeding if the inflow is not completely tied while the backflow is blocked. The inflow may be incompletely tied due to high arterial pressure or thick liver parenchym; the backflow, on the other hand, can be easily tied because of low pressure in the hepatic vein. In such situation, the ligature of the outflow should be released or severed, and immediately replaced with an untied suture. After dividing the main Glissonian pedicle of the inflow, the untied suture of the backflow is then secured.

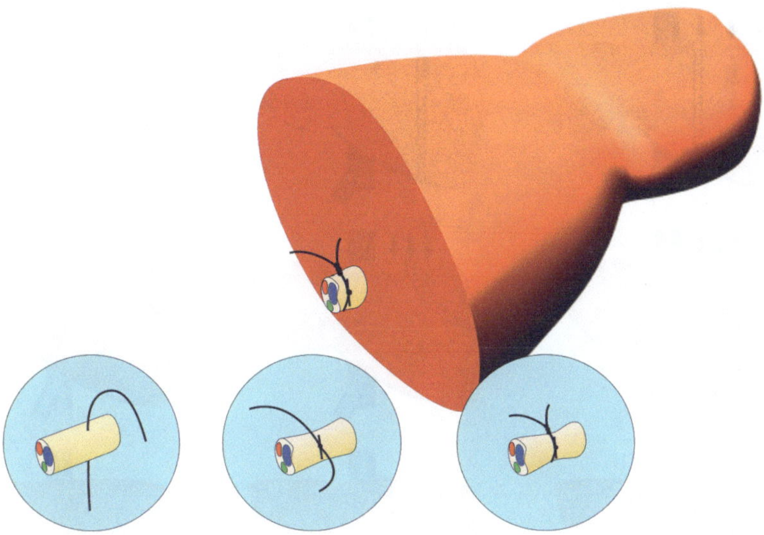

Fig. 2.5 Reinforcement of suture-ligation of the Glissonian pedicle

2.4 Typical Indications of the Straight Chang's Needle

Current indications for using the straight Chang's needle in hepatic resections are right lobectomy, S6 + 7 + 8 trisegmentectomy, left lateral segmentectomy, S7 + 8 or S5 + 6 bisegmentectomy, S2 or 3 segmentectomy of Couinaud classification, or nonanatomic resections shown in Fig. 2.6. Figure 2.7 shows our 102 hepatic resections, including a case with hepatorrhaphy.

The resections can be designed freely if the biliary drainage and hepatic inflow of the remnant liver can be properly preserved. Oblique puncture may also be used for lesions where vertical puncture is impossible [e.g., above the inferior vena cava (IVC)] using the straight needle. Currently, a curved needle is being developed to overcome such problems as well as to secure the inflow and outflow before laparoscopic liver resection. Severe liver laceration may also be easily suture-compressed using this needle.

A contraindication for the straight needle is tumors near or over the IVC.

2.5 Clinical Results

There were 66 HCCs, 5 cholangiocarcinomas (CCC), 10 colon metastases, 1 angiomyolipoma, 4 hemangiomas, 1 liver trauma, and 15 intrahepatic duct (IHD) stones. Thirty-five patients had mild to severe degrees of liver cirrhosis, and six patients had chronic active hepatitis. The remaining 61 patients had a normal liver.

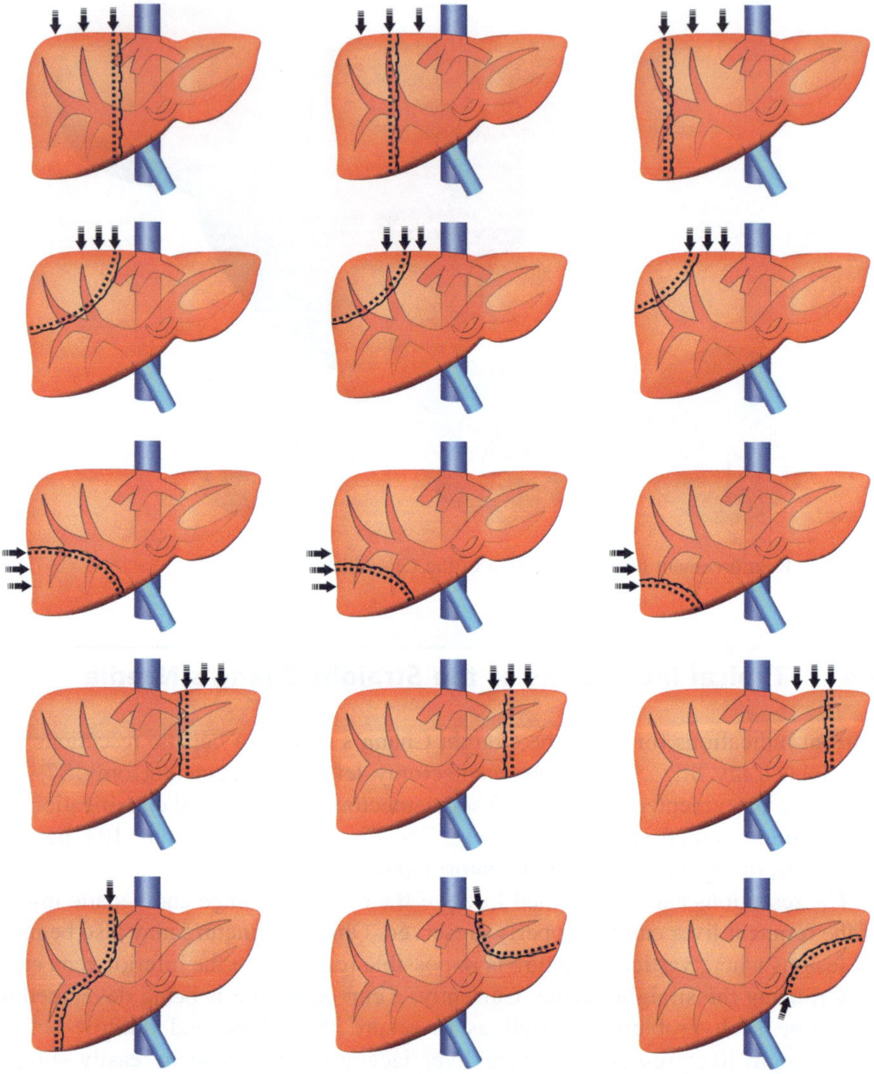

Fig. 2.6 Typical indications for straight Chang's needle

However, in two of the four patients with CCC, one liver showed marked cholestasis, while the other showed signs of sepsis before the operation. Chang's needle was used for hepatic resections in 13 right lobectomies, 3 trisegmentectomies, 25 bisegmentectomies, 17 segmentectomies, 20 subsegmentectomies, 5 wedge hepatectomies, 18 left lateral segmentectomies, and 1 hepatorrhaphy (Fig. 2.7). There was no procedure-related mortality. One patient had severe multiple injuries from a motor vehicle accident and died of multiorgan failure

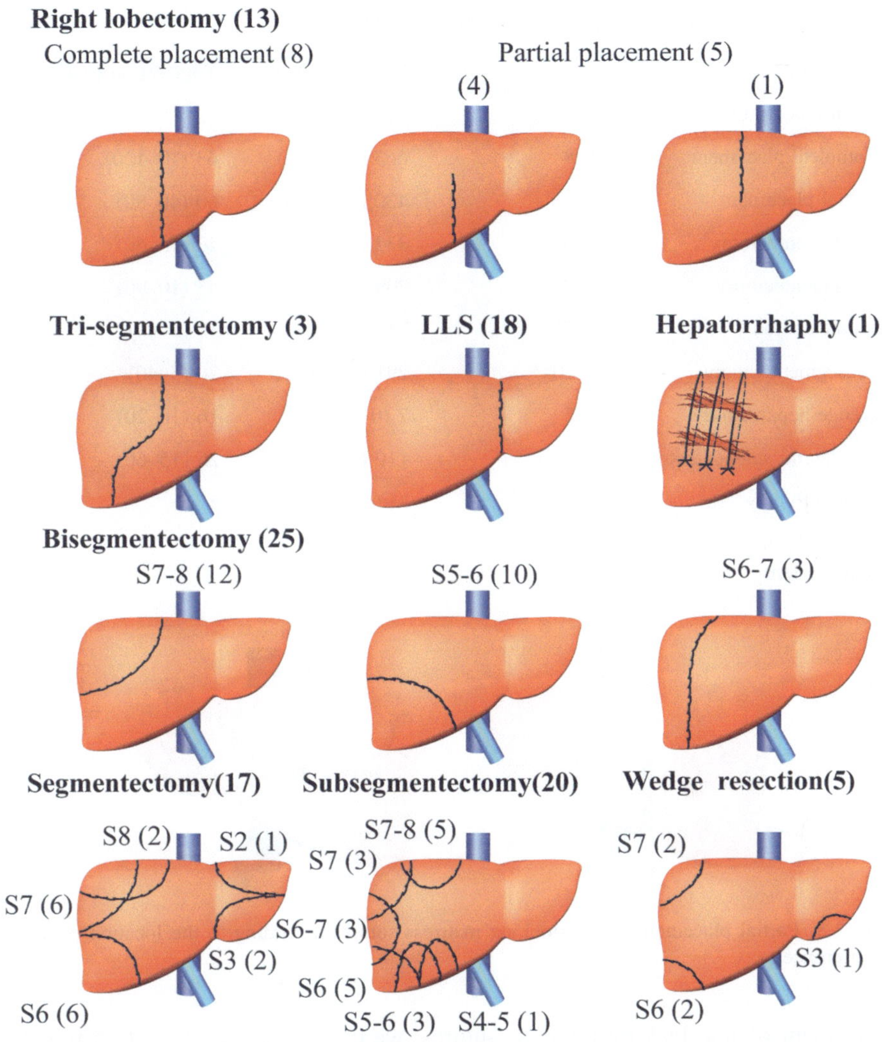

Fig. 2.7 102 clinical cases of straight Chang's needle

despite successful hemostasis for her liver laceration. Another died from severe nosocomial pneumonia [methicillin-resistant *Staphylococcus aureus* (MRSA)]. Minor bile leakage occurred in one case (1 %), but healed spontaneously. Three had hemorrhages; one minor hemorrhage stopped spontaneously, but the other two needed re-intervention, one of which was not attributable to the use of Chang's needle. Several patients with IHD stones experienced minor wound infections as a result of contamination from pus discharged from the bile duct. In most cases, only minimal hemorrhage was encountered during hepatic transection. The average durations of hepatic transections (Table 2.1), including the time required for

Table 2.1 102 hepatic resections using Chang's needle

Operation	Case number	Blood loss (ml)	Transection time (min)
Right lobectomy	13	612 (0–2,100)	62 (10–120)
Complete placement	8	663 (0–2,100)	63 (10–120)
Partial placement	5	430 (0–1,500)	60 (40–80)
Trisegmentectomy[a]	3	333 (0–700)	40 (15–60)
Bisegmentectomy	25	299 (0–1,950)	45 (10–90)
Segmentectomy	17	71 (0–300)	19 (3–40)
Subsegmentectomy	20	291 (0–350)	20 (5–40)
Wedge hepatectomy	5	7 (0–35)	16 (10–20)
Left lateral segmentectomy	18	110 (0–1,000[b])	25 (15–60)
Hepatorrhaphy	1	Minimal	5

[a] S6 + 7 + 8
[b] DIC patient

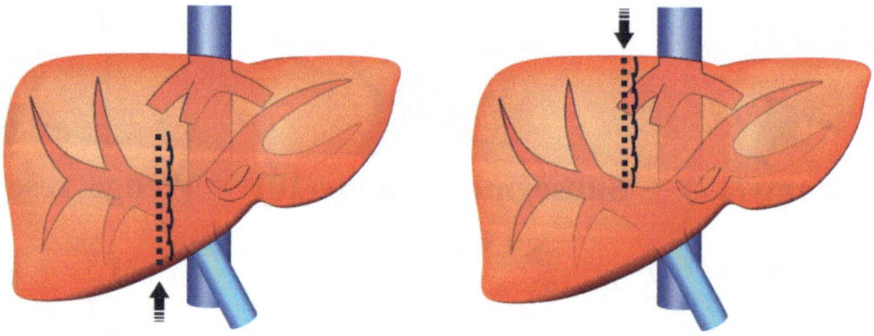

Fig. 2.8 Partial placement of interlocking mattress sutures according to the location of tumor interference

placement of interlocking mattress sutures, were 62, 40, 45, 19, and 25 min for right lobectomy, trisegmentectomy, bisegmentectomy, segmentectomy, and left lateral segmentectomy, respectively. It took only 5 min for hemostasis of liver laceration bleeding using compression sutures.

2.6 Partial Placement

Occasionally, tumors located near the IVC or the entrance of the right hepatic vein (Fig. 2.8, left), or near the bifurcation of the right portal vein (Fig. 2.8, right) will disturb complete placement of the interlocking mattress sutures. In the former case, partial placement can be done first, followed by conventional transection without using Pringle's maneuver [5]. In the latter case, hilar ligation of the vessels

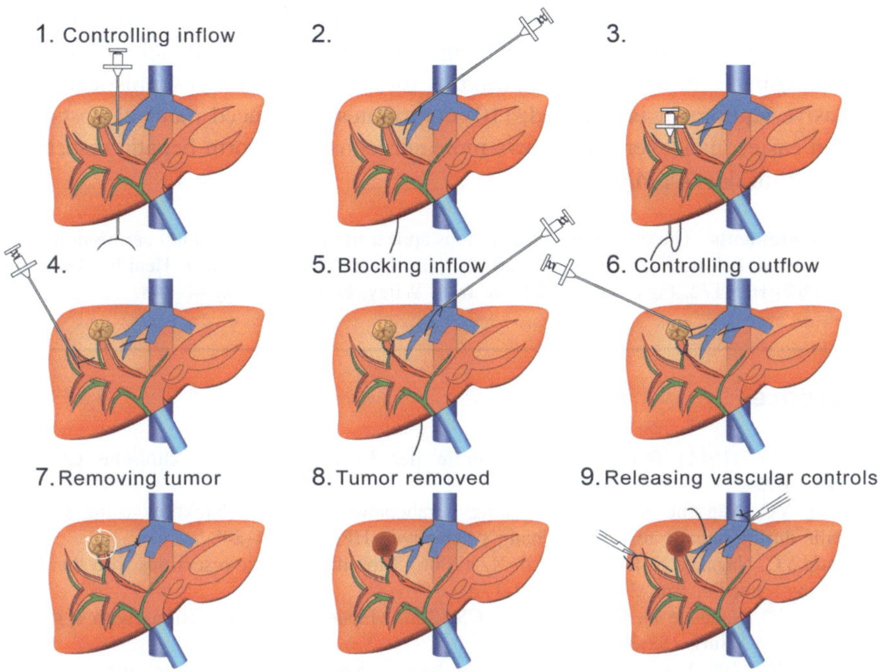

Fig. 2.9 Chang's maneuver for selective, temporary, or permanent blocking of intrahepatic inflow and backflow

and bile duct and conventional transection can be done before partial placement of the interlocking mattress sutures.

2.7 Chang's Maneuver: Selective, Temporary, or Permanent Blocking of Intrahepatic Inflow and Backflow

Intraoperative ultrasound (with or without Doppler function) is used to locate the respective inflow and backflow vessels, and then Chang's maneuver is used on these vessels (Fig. 2.9) before starting the hepatic resection. After the resection, the inflow and backflow blocks may be released.

2.8 Advantages of the Current Technique

The advantages of this maneuver can be summarized as follows: (1) inexpensive, simple, and reusable instruments are used; (2) Pringle's maneuver is unnecessary; (3) shortened operation time; (4) fewer or no blood transfusions needed in most cases; (5) fibrin glue is unnecessary; (6) fewer ischemic and reperfusion injuries of the remnant liver, which leads to simpler postoperative care; (7) a lower level of stress for the surgeon during parenchyma transection due to the lack of bleeding; (8) less demand for technique and training for surgeons; (9) less sophisticated and expensive equipment is required; (10) contributes to reduced medical costs; and (11) an easier maneuver that allows more surgeons to perform hepatic resections, especially in developing countries.

Acknowledgments The undernoted illustrations appear in this chapter by kind permission of the sources listed below: Figs. 2.1, 2.6, and 2.7 are from Wolters Kluwer Health, Ann Surg 2006;243(2):169–172. Figs. 2.2 and 2.9 are from Wiley, HPB 2008;10:244–248.

References

1. Wendel W (1911) Beiträge zur Chirurgie der Leber. Archiv für klinische Chirurgie 95:887–895
2. Chang YC, Nagasue N (2008) Blocking intrahepatic inflow and backflow using Chang's needle during hepatic resection: Chang's maneuver. HPB 10:244–248
3. Chang YC, Nagasue N, Chen CS, Lin XZ (2006) Simplified hepatic resections with the use of a Chang's needle. Ann Surg 243:169–172
4. Chang YC, Nagasue N, Lin XZ, Chen CS (2001) Easier hepatic resections with a straight needle. Am J Surg 182:260–264
5. Pringle JG (1908) Notes on the arrest of hepatic hemorrhage due to trauma. Ann Surg 48:541–549

Open Hepatic Transection Using PMOD

3

Shu You Peng, Jiang Tao Li and Zhi Jian Tan

3.1 Introduction

There are a great variety of techniques for liver parenchymal transection, including the finger fracture method, clamp-crush technique, cavitron ultrasonic surgical aspirator (CUSA), water jet (WJ), TissueLink, LigaSure, harmonic scalpel, microwave sealer, Peng's multifunction operative dissector (PMOD), radiofrequency sealer, and vascular stapler [1–3].

According to their function, all these devices/techniques may be divided into two groups: (I) for precise dissection (of the ductal system across the transection plane) and (II) for precoagulation (of the liver parenchymal transection plane).

Electronic Supplementary Material The online version of this article (doi: 10.1007/978-88-470-2622-3_3) contains supplementary material, which is available to authorized users.

S. Y. Peng (✉) · J. T. Li
Department of Surgery, Second Affiliated Hospital, Zhejiang University Medical School, Hangzhou, Zhejiang, People's Republic of China
e-mail: zrwkpsy@163.com

J. T. Li
e-mail: zjuljt@gmail.com

S. Y. Peng
Department of Surgery, Sir Run Run Shaw Hospital, Zhejiang University Medical School, Hangzhou, Zhejiang, People's Republic of China

Z. J. Tan
Department of Surgery, Second Affiliated Hospital, Guangzhou University of Chinese Medicine, Guangzhou, Guangdong, People's Republic of China
e-mail: doctortan@vip.sina.com

I. Di Carlo (ed.), *Open, Laparoscopic and Robotic Hepatic Transection*, DOI: 10.1007/978-88-470-2622-3_3, © Springer-Verlag Italia 2012

Those belonging to group I are the finger fracture method, clamp-crush technique, PMOD, CUSA, and WJ, while the rest belong to group II.

Precise dissection and precoagulation are two different functions. By using the instruments that belong to group I, all the vessels/bile ducts along the transection plane can be isolated and dealt with individually so as to achieve precise dissection.

By using the instruments that belong to group II, the transection plane is pre-coagulated or prestapled before the transection plane is directly cut into. This may be called blind transection, which is very good for peripheral liver resection yet not good for central liver resection that requires precise dissection.

Essentially, all the above-mentioned devices can perform only one of the functions, i.e., either dissection or precoagulation (clip-close the vessels when it comes to the the vascular stapler technique). However, the PMOD is the only instrument that can perform both functions.

Being a versatile device, it is called a multifunction operative dissector.

3.2 Device Description

Peng's multifunction operative dissector (PMOD) [Hangzhou Shuyou Medical Instrument Co, Hangzhou, Zhejiang, PR China; FDA 510(K) number K040780] is a special instrument with the functions of dissection, electrocutting, electrocoagulation, curetting, and aspiration, separately or synchronously, so that the surgical field can be kept clear and clean. The best aspect of the PMOD is that it can delineate all the vessels and ductal system so that the intrahepatic ductal structures can be identified, isolated, and treated individually.

The PMOD looks like an electrosurgical pencil, but their structures are different. The main difference is that a metal pipe passes through the pencil, while the body of the pipe is coated with insulated material and the tip of the pipe is made oblique, forming a bevel end. A removable blade is attached to the tip of the tube for electric cutting. This special design enables the PMOD to offer four different functions (Figs. 3.1, 3.2). The pipe is connected to a vacuum apparatus through a tube. The PMOD also has an electric wire to connect with a regular electrosurgical generator.

Both the aspiration tube and wire are anchored onto the operating table by the right side of surgeon, with a length of 60–80 cm free so that the surgeon can manipulate the PMOD conveniently (Fig. 3.3).

3.3 Technique Description

PMOD is used to scrape (curettage) on the liver incision line. Debris and oozing blood, if any, are sucked away synchronously, so as to expose and deal with the vessels and bile ducts individually in the parenchyma. Therefore, this dissection technique is termed "curettage and aspiration dissection technique" (CADT) [4, 5].

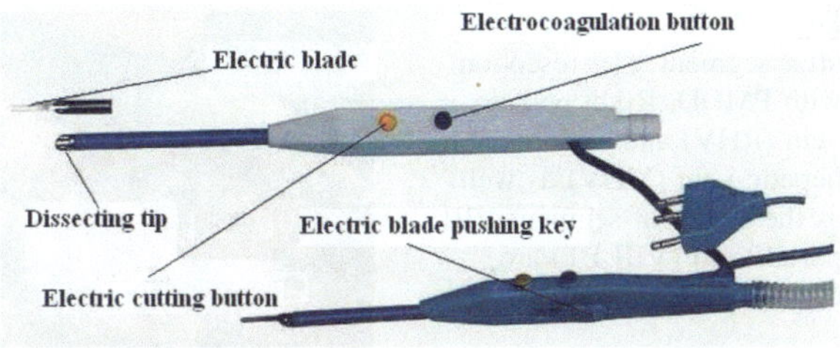

Fig. 3.1 A different side view of the PMOD, a removable blade is attached to the tip of the tube for electric cutting

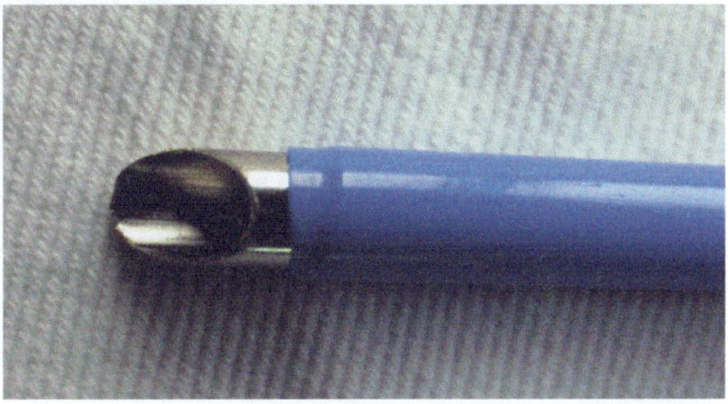

Fig. 3.2 A bevel end design enables the PMOD to offer four different functions

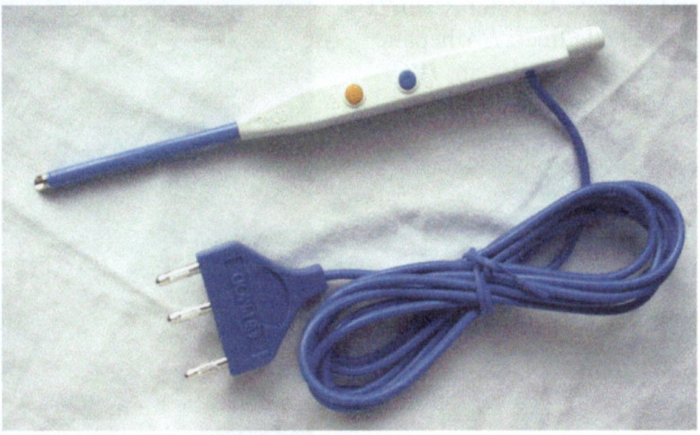

Fig. 3.3 Overview of PMOD

The PMOD is held in the hand just like a pen. By using the thumb or index finger to control the "on" or "off" button, tissue can be dissected with the bevel edge of the tip.

During mechanically scraping and dissecting, the tip is essentially not electrified. Blood, fluid, and oddment in the operative field can be aspirated away continually to make the operating field clear and clean [6–9].

The CADT maneuver is composed of four principal surgical actions: curettage, aspiration, electrocoagulation, and dissection by use of PMOD.

PMOD allows the operator to perform all operative manipulations (except suturing), including cutting, hemostasis, suction, and dissection, so as to avoid the necessity of changing surgical instruments frequently. As a result, operating time and

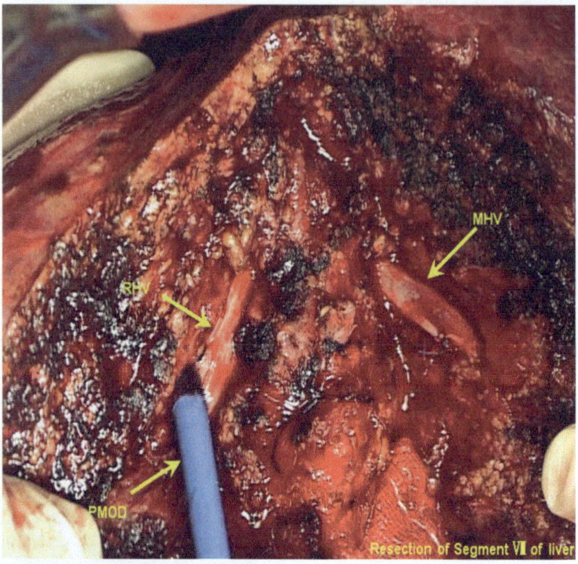

Fig. 3.4 Raw surface seen after segment VIII resection with PMOD. Right hepatic vein (RHV) and middle hepatic vein (MHV) as well as the stump of segment VIII portal traid (VIII PT) are clearly shown

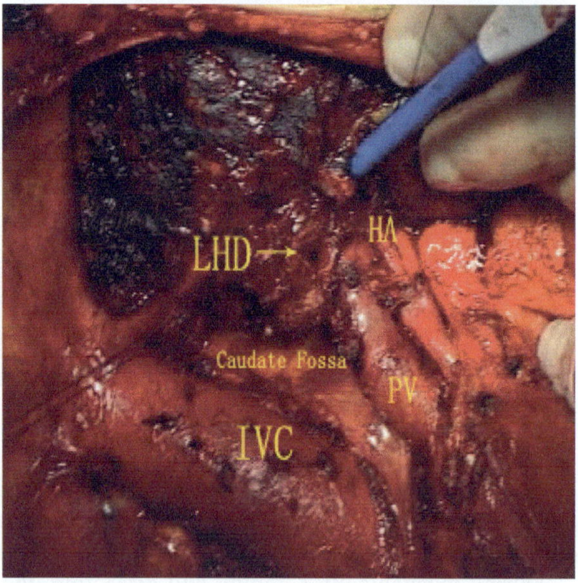

Fig. 3.5 View after right and caudate lobectomy. *LHD* left hepatic duct, *HA* hepatic artery, *PV* portal vein, *IVC* inferior vena cava

blood loss are reduced and the quality of operation is improved. These manipulations can be performed simultaneously or in sequence (Figs. 3.4, 3.5, 3.6, 3.7).

During liver resection, intermittent inflow occlusion is routinely used; the time limit is 10 min each time, with 2 min reperfusion. Total vascular exclusion is seldom necessary except when the tumor is closely adherent to the IVC or major hepatic veins. In some cases, the major hepatic vein (right hepatic vein and/or

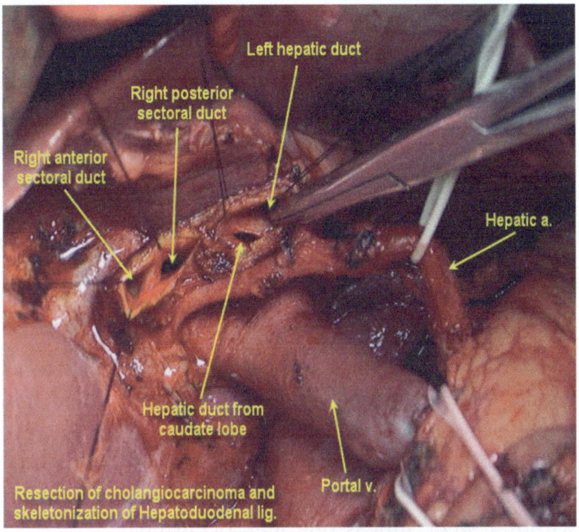

Fig. 3.6 Resection of cholangiocarcinoma and skeletonization of hepatoduodenal ligament with PMOD

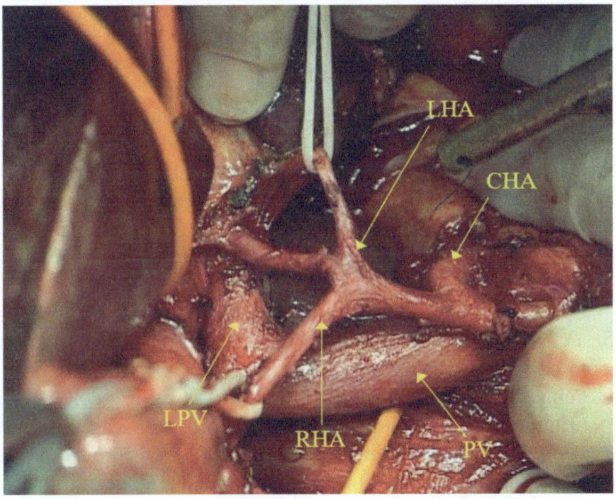

Fig. 3.7 Skeletonization of hepatoduodenal ligament in hilar cholangiocarcinoma radical resection. *LHA* left hepatic artery, *CHA* common hepatic artery, *PV* portal vein, *RPV* right portal vein, *RHA* right hepatic artery, *LPV* left portal vein

common trunk of middle and left hepatic veins) are dissected and prelooped with tape to substitute IVC control.

The power setting of the electrosurgical generator used varies according to the tissue to be dissected or transected. For dissection and division of hepatic ligament, 40–60 Hz is sufficient. For liver parenchyma, a maximum power of 120 Hz can be appropriate.

Liver capsule is cut before CADT starts. The strength of scraping varies with the texture of the liver. When the liver is soft, gentle scraping is enough. If the liver is cirrhotic, the scraping strength may need to be increased.

Dissection also can be achieved by using the bevel to push liver tissue to both sides.

Usually, dissection is carried out along the transection plane, yet when large vessel is encountered, curettage proceeds in parenchyma parallel to the vessel by altering the scraping direction, so as to expose a short segment of the vessel for division and ligation/clipping or coagulation. It is advisable to coagulate a short segment of the vessel for secure hemostasis. To prevent blockage of the aspirating portion of PMOD, it is advisable to aspirate blood with the bevel before twisting 180° to coagulate with the back of the tip.

Hepatic vein tributaries up to 3 mm in diameter can be coagulated, but the Glissonian tributaries should be ligated when the diameter is larger than 1 mm.

Tension should be kept by fingers or stay sutures on both sides of the tissue to be dissected to facilitate the transection process.

Two PMODs can also be used at the same time, separately held by two surgeons, to expedite the process of dissection and homeostasis.

After resection, the cut surface of liver is generally electrocoagulated with PMOD. Bleeding points may be sutured with 4-0 or 5-0 prolene. Bile leak is examined and treated when identified. Drains are routinely placed and removed within 1 week unless bile leak occurred.

References

1. Pamecha V, Gurusamy KS, Sharma D, Davidson BR (2009) Techniques for liver parenchymal transection: a meta-analysis of randomized controlled trials. HPB (Oxford). 11(4):275–281
2. Rau HG, Schardey HM, Buttler E et al. (1995) A comparison of different techniques for liver resection: blunt dissection, ultrasonic aspirator and jet-cutter. Eur J Surg Oncol 21:183–187
3. Topp SA, McClurken M, Lipson D et al. (2004) Saline-linked surface radiofrequency ablation: factors affecting steam popping and depth of injury in the pig liver. Ann Surg 239:518–527
4. Di Carlo I (2007) Peng's Multifunctional Operational Dissector (PMOD). In: Chirurgia Epatica. Edizioni Minerva Medica: 34–35
5. Peng SY, Li JT (2008) "Curettage and aspiration dissection technique" using PMOD for liver resection. HPB (Oxford) 10(4): 285–288
6. Peng SY, Li JT, Liu YB et al. (2006) Surgical treatment of hepatocellular carcinoma originating from caudate lobe—a report of 39 cases. J Gastrointest Surg 10(3):371–378
7. Peng SY, Li JT, Mou YP et al. (2003) Different approaches to caudate lobectomy with "curettage and aspiration" technique using a special instrument PMOD: a report of 76 cases. World J Gastroenterol 9(10):2169–2173
8. Peng SY, Jiang XC, Li JD, Cai XJ, Peng CH, Mou YP, Su Y, Fan MM (1995) Liver transection by curettage and aspiration—A new technique for hepatectomy (in Chinese). J Basic Clin Gen Surg 2:11–13
9. Ji ZL, Peng SY, Cai XJ (2004) A laparoscopic multifunctional operative device in laparoscopic hepatectomy. Chir Gastroenterol 20(4):308–312

Open Hepatic Transection Using Dissecting Sealer

4

Isidoro Di Carlo and Adriana Toro

4.1 Introduction

Procedures for liver transection have been improved gradually and progressively in the last decades. The main focus of technical innovation has been to decrease intraoperative bleeding, which may increase morbidity and mortality. Tissue coagulation using electrical energy is the most widespread method used for coagulation, but unfortunately in liver parenchyma is not safe for liver transection due to eschar formation and related complications. To avoid these complications and for improved local action, at the beginning of 2000, a water-cooled high-frequency monopolar device named Floating Ball was developed for open surgery by TissueLink Medical Inc., Dover, NH, USA. Currently, this device has been replaced by two different devices named Dissecting Sealer (DS 3.0 and 3.5-C) by Salient Surgical Technologies, Dover, NH, USA. The mechanism of action is the same for all three devices, the difference being only in the aspect of the tip (Fig. 4.1). The aim of this chapter is to describe the cited devices for open surgery and the related technique.

Electronic Supplementary Material The online version of this article (doi: 10.1007/978-88-470-2622-3_4) contains supplementary material which is available to authorized users.

I. Di Carlo (✉) · A. Toro
Department of Surgical Sciences, Organ Transplantation and Advanced Technologies, University of Catania, Cannizzaro Hospital, Catania, Italy
e-mail: idicarlo@unict.it

A. Toro
e-mail: atoroct@gmail.com

I. Di Carlo (ed.), *Open, Laparoscopic and Robotic Hepatic Transection*,
DOI: 10.1007/978-88-470-2622-3_4, © Springer-Verlag Italia 2012

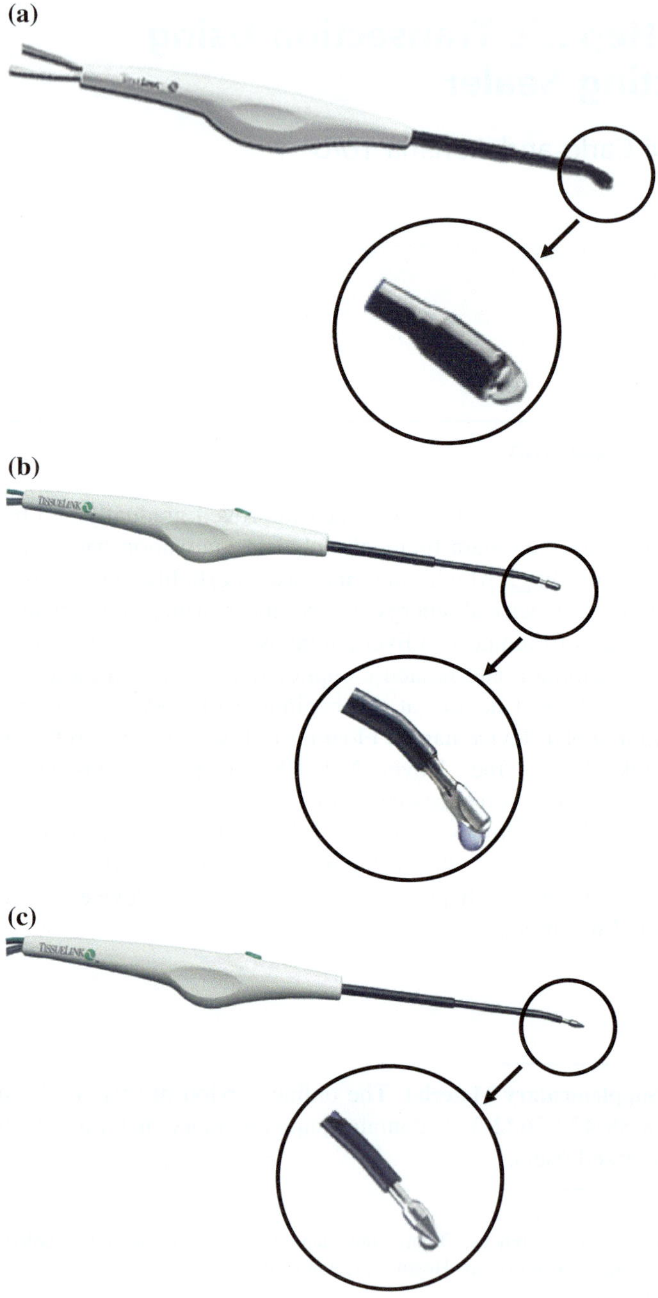

Fig. 4.1 Different types of the device. From *top* to *bottom*: **a** Floating Ball, **b** dissecting sealer, **c** Cone Tip

4.2 Device Description

The dissecting sealer (DS) is a sterile, single-use monopolar electrosurgical device with a power cord that connects to a standard electrocautery generator for delivery of radiofrequency (RF) power as well as a fluid pathway that exits the tip of the device and connects to a 1-l bag of sterile saline solution. The generator used is usually set to 80 W (range 50–100 W), and the device should be slowly applied against the tissue to ensure the proper generator setting and saline drip rate (usually one drop per second). Use of a return electrode plate is required for this device. If saline solution stops during the electrosurgical procedure, use of the device should be stopped and attempts made to resume the saline flow. The saline source should be adequate, and the saline delivery system has to function properly. If the saline flow cannot be restabilized, use of the DS should be suspended and a new line should be initiated.

The device has a proximal and a distal end, comprising: a handle; a button in the middle of the superior part of the handle; extending from the handle, a shaft supporting an electrode tip in rigid relation to the handle and having a distal end; a fluid passage being connectable to a fluid source.

The electrode tip comprises a single metal contact element providing an electrode with a distal portion and a proximal portion; the distal portion of the electrode extends distally beyond the distal end of the shaft, the proximal portion of the electrode being contained within the shaft. The distal portion of the electrode has length of 11.43 mm and diameter of 3.5 mm. At the end of the tip, there is an angle of 10°. Finally, the length of the shaft outside of the body is 110.5 mm.

The distal portion of the electrode comprises an electrically conductive cone-shaped portion, having a circular portion which narrows towards the distal end of the device along an electrically conductive cone-shaped surface (Fig. 4.2).

One fluid outlet opening in fluid communication with the fluid passage is located at the distal end of the shaft, adjacent to the electrode. This distal portion of the device is designed to provide radiofrequency power and fluid simultaneously. Finally, the button positioned at the top of the middle portion of the handle permits activation of the device function.

4.3 Technique Description

The water-cooled high-frequency monopolar device (DS) for parenchymal transection is a surgical instrument that couples radiofrequency energy (480 kHz) with conductive fluid. Electrical energy is conducted through a continuous low-volume (4–6 ml/min) flow of 0.9 % saline solution dripping from the tip and then into tissue, where it is converted into heat by ohmic heating of the tissue. The saline facilitates energy transfer across the device–tissue interface, maintaining contact with the hepatic tissue and dispersing thermal energy [1]. Coagulation of liver tissue is achieved by denaturation of intramolecular crosslinks of triple-helix

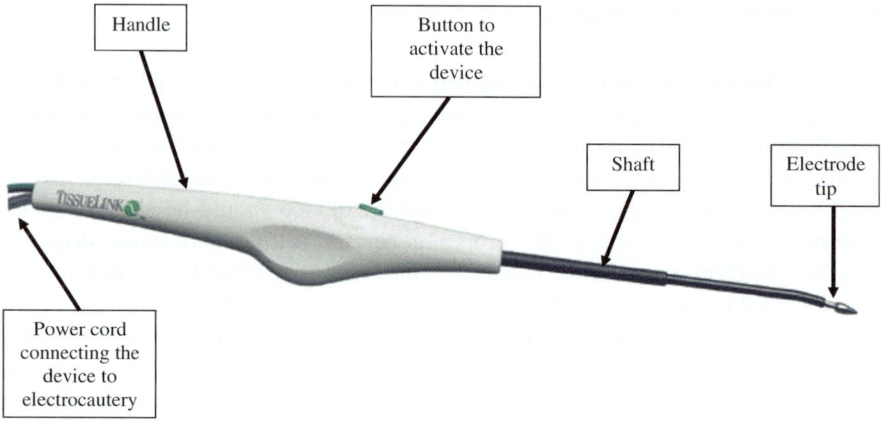

Fig. 4.2 Framework of the devices

proteic structures, keeping the temperature of liver surface below 100 °C to avoid development of eschar [2]. As a result, vessels <3 mm are sealed through shrinkage of collagen, and their lumens are stably occluded. Larger structures remain isolated and can be tied or clipped during parenchymal transection performed with Kelly forceps or other tools. Hepatic tissue coagulated without eschar is softer, more friable, and easier to dissect than tissue that has been charred at higher temperature [1]. In contrast, in electrocautery the tissue temperature rises above 300 °C, which causes dessication and fragility of the tissue. Hepatic resection using DS would therefore be expected to yield more stable hemostasis. The device can be used both for precoagulation of the liver parenchyma before transecting it or to coagulate the surface after transection without precoagulation. In the former case the tip of the DS 3.5-C is more useful, whereas in the second case the DS 3.0 is the most used tool, although both devices can be used for either procedure. The following description is the personal technique used by the authors to perform hepatic resection.

The first step of the procedure is echographic examination of the liver to confirm the preoperative diagnosis concerning the number and location of liver tumors. Thereafter, the part of the liver that is to be resected is gently delimited on the Glisson surface using common electrocautery. Subsequently, the DS is introduced into the hepatic parenchyma and activated. The device is left in situ until the liver parenchyma up to 1 cm around the tip changes color, indicating that precoagulation of the hepatic parenchyma has been achieved to a distance (outward and downwards) of 1 cm (Fig. 4.3). This device does not cause eschar formation, so extracting it does not produce bleeding. The device is then moved 1 cm ahead, and the maneuver is repeated. At the end of coagulation of the traced line, a small Kelly forceps is used to fracture the liver parenchyma. In this way, only vessels larger than 3 mm remain to be identified and clipped or ligated and cut; the smallest vessels have already been coagulated. Once the first line of hepatic

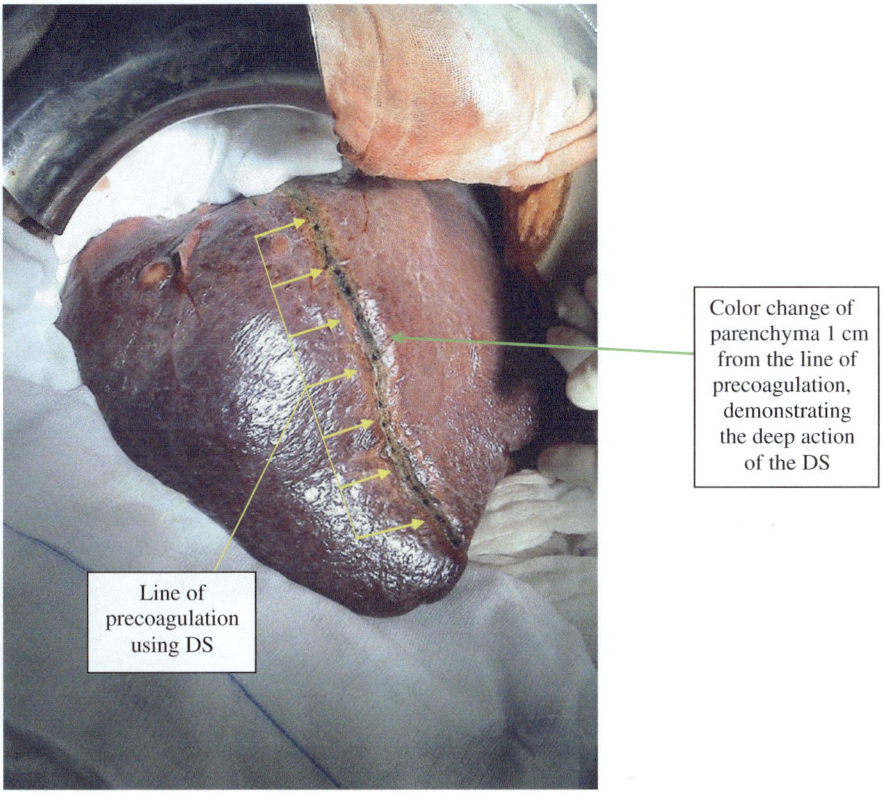

Fig. 4.3

parenchyma treated with the DS has been opened, the maneuver is repeated until the resection is complete (Figs. 4.4, 4.5).

Usually in this technique no Pringle maneuver is required; in case of bleeding, simple bimanual parenchymal compression may help to stop the bleeding [3]. Differently from many techniques described in literature, we perform transection using the Kelly clamp after precoagulation. In effect, transection with the DS is possible, but in the superficial part of the liver parenchyma. In this part, there are no vessels or biliary structures larger than 3 mm. However, when the resection becomes deeper, transection with the DS is not possible due to the presence of larger vessels that are not suitable for treatment with DS. In this way, precoagulation and transection of the liver with Kelly clamp permits safe and bloodless transection, avoiding damage to large vessels by DS and consequent intraoperative hemorrhage [4].

The benefits of this technique have not been widely confirmed, but many studies have demonstrated that use of DS has a beneficial effect with respect to blood loss and reperfusion-related liver injury, which is particularly useful in

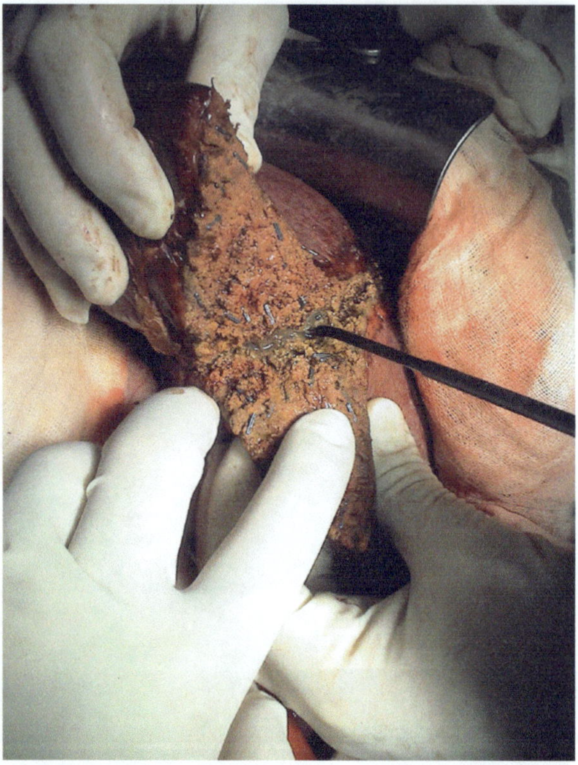

Fig. 4.4 Using the same procedure, all the liver parenchyma can be precoagulated

cirrhotic patients [5, 6]. In fact, the conventional approach to liver transection using a crushing clamp without precoagulation requires Pringle's maneuver to reduce intraoperative blood loss.

The only disadvantage of this device is represented by the prolonged time needed to perform the hepatic transection. Consequently, the procedure needs more patience and skill by the operator because heavy bleeding may occur if the parenchyma is dissected before the small vessels are properly coagulated [7].

The cost of the device may vary between countries and high- and low-volume centers. However, a reliable cost analysis between the DS and other devices is not currently possible owing to the different costs of the system consoles, disposable parts, and maintenance of different devices [8].

Moreover, use of DS is associated with less use of hemostatic agents. In fact, the DS is based on RF energy that heats and coagulates the surrounding parenchyma, whereas other devices such as ultrasound or water-jet devices, fragment, irrigate, and aspirate the liver tissue without coagulation. This may explain the increased use of stapler of hemostatic agents when ultrasound or water jet are used.

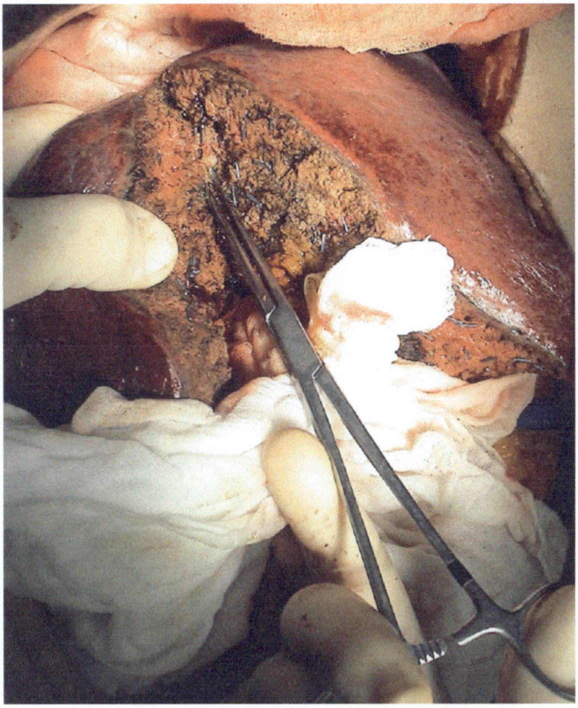

Fig. 4.5 Structures (vessel or biliary duct) larger than 3 mm have to be ligated or clipped before division

Finally, the DS when applied for longer on the surface of in situ margin after resection of a tumor, could induce a pronounced heat-zone area, inside which cells (including possible remaining tumoral cells) could be efficiently destroyed [9].

References

1. Di Carlo I, Barbagallo F, Toro A, Sofia M, Guastella T, Latteri F (2004) Hepatic resection using a water-cooled, high-density, monopolar device: a new technology for safer surgery. J Gastroint Surg 8:596–600
2. Furrer K, De Oliveira ML, Graf R, Clavien PA (2007) Improving out come in patients undergoing liver surgery. Liver Int 27:26–39
3. Di Carlo I, Pulvirenti E, Guastella T, Toro A (2011) Parenchymal compression and new devices for hepatic resections: re-visitation of an old technique. Hepatogastroenterology 58:980–983
4. Di Carlo I, Pulvirenti E, Toro A (2008) Use of dissecting sealer may affect the early outcome in patients submitted to hepatic resection. HPB (Oxf) 10:271–274
5. Fan ST, Lai EC, Lo CM, Ng IO, Wong J (1995) Hospital mortality of major hepatectomy for hepatocellular carcinoma associated with cirrhosis. Arch Surg 130:198–203
6. Sakamoto Y, Yamamoto J, Kokudo N, Seki M, Kosuge T, Yamaguchi T, Muto T, Makuuchi M (2004) Bloodless liver resection using the monopolar floating ball plus ligasure diathermy: preliminary results of 16 liver resections. World J Surg 28:166–172

7. Xia F, Wang S, Ma K, Feng X, Su Y, Dong J (2008) The use of saline-linked radiofrequency dissecting sealer for liver transection in patients with cirrhosis. J Surg Res 149:110–114
8. Richter S, Kollmar O, Schuld J, Moussavian MR, Igna D, Schilling MK (2009) Randomized clinical trial of efficacy and costs of three dissection devices in liver resection. Br J Surg 96:593–601
9. Kianmanesh R, Ogata S, Paradis V, Sauvanet A, Belghiti J (2008) Heat-zone effect after surface application of dissecting sealer on the "in situ margin" after tumorectomy for liver tumors. J Am Coll Surg 206:1122–1128

Open Hepatic Transection Using Habib™ 4X

5

Charis Kyriakides, Feng Xi, Madhava Pai and Nagy A. Habib

5.1 Introduction

Intraoperative blood loss, parenchymal sparing, and liver functional reserve are outlined as major independent predictive factors for surgical morbidity and mortality after liver resection [1]. Radiofrequency (RF)-assisted liver surgery remains today the only surgical technique that reduces blood loss while maximizing parenchymal sparing, with reduced or even no liver warm ischemia. RF was initially designed for local ablation of unresectable solid tumors as a means of palliation. In recent years, use of RF has been introduced to the area of curative surgery in liver resection. RF is used to create a plane of coagulative necrosis tissue along the intended line of parenchymal transection. In early experience, this kind of RF-assisted liver resection was performed using monopolar RF devices

Electronic Supplementary Material The online version of this article (doi:10.1007/978-88-470-2622-3_5) contains supplementary material which is available to authorized users.

N. A. Habib (✉) · C. Kyriakides · F. Xi · M. Pai
HPB Surgery, Hammersmith Hospital, Imperial College London, London, UK
e-mail: nagy.habib@imperial.ac.uk

C. Kyriakides
e-mail: charis.kyriakides@imperial.nhs.uk

F. Xi
e-mail: Feng.xi.cn@gmail.com

M. Pai
e-mail: madhava.pai@imperial.ac.uk

I. Di Carlo (ed.), *Open, Laparoscopic and Robotic Hepatic Transection*,
DOI: 10.1007/978-88-470-2622-3_5, © Springer-Verlag Italia 2012

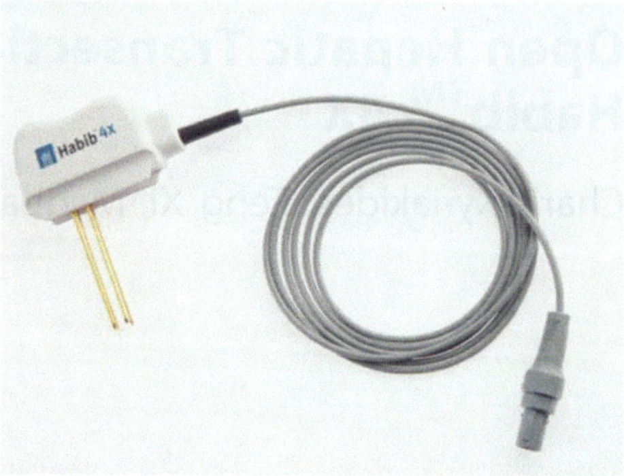

Fig. 5.1 Habib 4X bipolar radiofrequency device

primarily designed for tumor ablation, which released an uncontrolled amount of energy and produced excessive amount of tissue necrosis with the potential risk of septic complications. Research on enhancing the use of this power source for liver resection led to the development of a bipolar, handheld, disposable RF device known as the Habib™ 4X. This bipolar RF device releases controlled RF energy between two pairs of electrodes, producing a plane of coagulative necrosis along the intended line of parenchymal transection. It is an effective, minimal blood loss surgical technique, with no need of hepatic pedicle clamping, total vascular exclusion, or hypotensive anesthetics.

5.2 Device Description

Habib™ 4X (AngioDynamics Inc., Queensbury, NY, USA) is a bipolar, handheld, disposable RF device that can be used in conjunction with the RITA1500/1500X generator. It consists of two pairs of opposing electrodes with an active end of 6 or 10 cm in length (Fig. 5.1). The device is connected to a 500-kHz generator (model 1500X; AngioDynamics Inc., Queensbury, NY, USA) which produces up to 250 W of RF power. It allows measurement of the generator output, tissue impedance, temperature, and time of application. The system also includes a pneumatic foot pedal used to turn the RF energy on and off. The generator can be run in manual or automatic mode. On connecting the device and switching on the generator, the RF power setting defaults to 125 W, and this can be modified according to user experience and the thermal requirement of the individual tissue types.

5.3 Operative Technique

After laparotomy, a careful search is performed for local recurrence, and extra-hepatic and peritoneal disease. Any suspicious lesions are examined by frozen section. Intraoperative bimanual liver palpation and ultrasonography are then performed to confirm tumor location and size. Extensive liver mobilization is

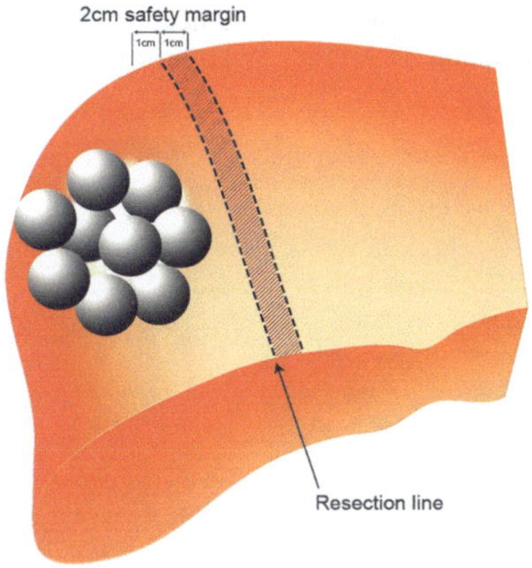

Fig. 5.2 Line of resection marked after intraoperative ultrasound

avoided whenever possible, with only the side to be resected being mobilized in most cases. Cholecystectomy is not routinely performed unless the proposed transection line involves the gallbladder fossa. Formal hilar dissection is seldom performed, with vascular clamping being required in only two of our cases. Hilar dissection was only done when the tumor was adjacent (1 cm or less) to the hepatic hilum. In these cases, separation of the tumor from the hilar structures is achieved by dissection and ligation of the ipsilateral arterial and portal vessels prior to application of the probe, thus avoiding injury to the contralateral hilar structures. Similarly, dissection of the hepatic veins is not performed routinely unless the tumor is in close proximity. In these cases, dissection and ligation of the hepatic vein are completed before application of the probe to avoid injury to the inferior vena cava (IVC).

After the tumor localization, the resection line is marked with argon diathermy, 1 cm from the edge of the tumor (Fig. 5.2). Clearly marking the transection line prior to resection is important, as following RF application the hepatic parenchyma undergoes coagulative necrosis and hardens, which makes palpation of the tumor edge difficult and interferes with intraoperative ultrasound (IOUS) imaging.

Application of the Habib™ 4X to the liver parenchyma along the resection line was done in the following steps:

1. The device was introduced perpendicularly into the liver, abutting the transection line (Fig. 5.3). The generator was programmed to produce an alert signal when energy delivery had been automatically stopped, thus avoiding overcoagulation and carbonation. The probe was gently moved to and fro in its vertical axis for 3–5 mm throughout the coagulation process to avoid adherence of the probe to liver parenchyma. The process took less than 1 min for each application in normal liver tissue. The probe was then reintroduced adjacent to the last coagulated area in serial fashion, until the area to be transected was fully ablated. The number of applications required to create a complete zone of desiccation was related to the size of the cut surface of the resection margin.

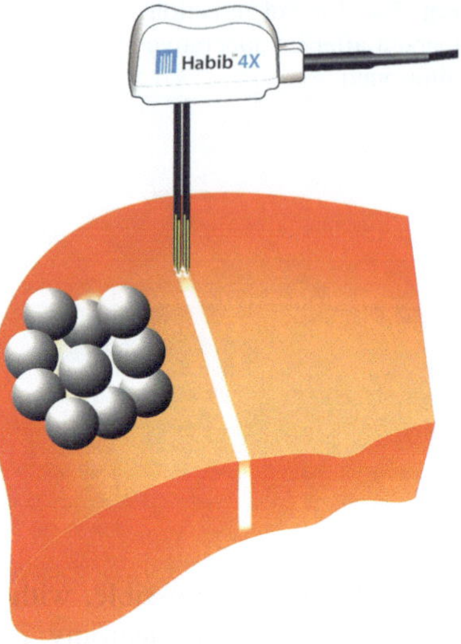

Fig. 5.3 First line of vertical ablation

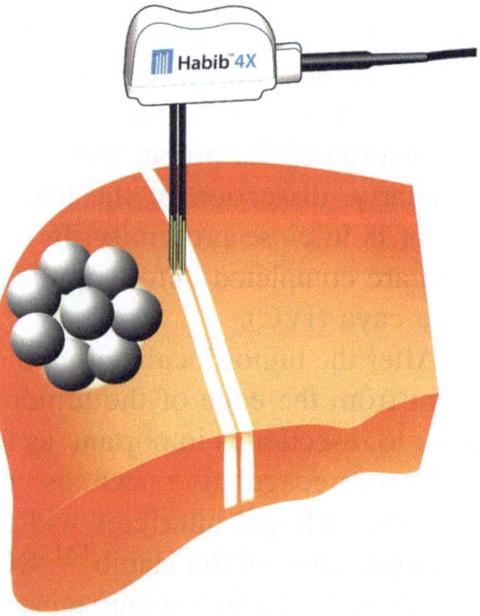

Fig. 5.4 Second line of vertical ablation

2. A second line of ablation, parallel to the first line and closer to the tumor edge, was then done to ensure complete tissue coagulation and perfect hemostasis prior to transection (Fig. 5.4).
3. The Habib^{TM} 4X was then applied perpendicularly to the previous two lines of ablation, so as to ensure complete coagulation of any residual normal liver parenchyma (Fig. 5.5). This allowed a margin of coagulated liver parenchyma to remain, ensuring vessels and bile ducts remained sealed. For deeper tumors the device was applied at an angle of 45° to the surface.
4. During liver transection itself, the device was again introduced. A scalpel was applied perpendicularly in order to divide the parenchyma along the pair of

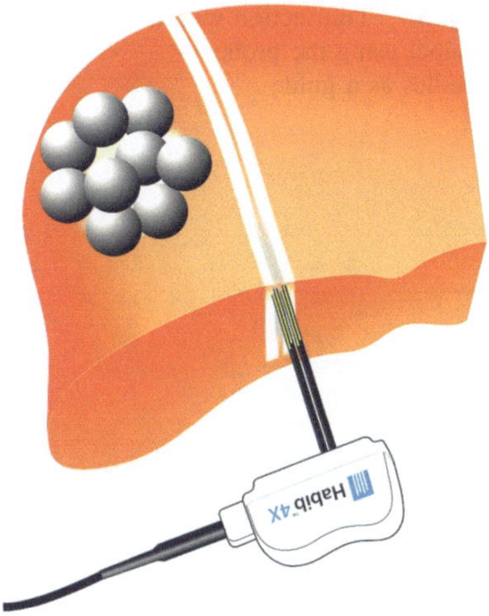

Fig. 5.5 Line of transverse ablation

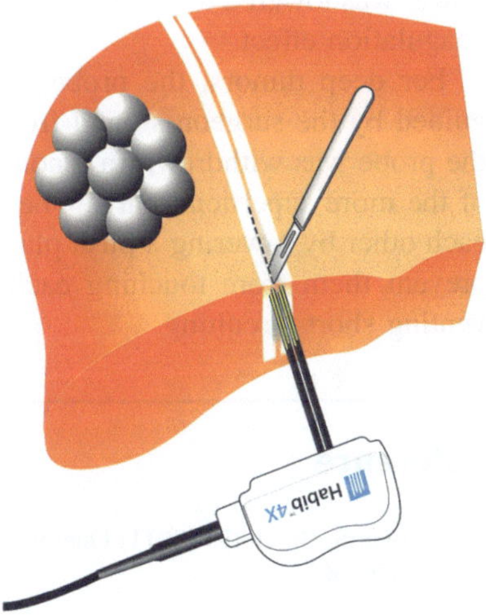

Fig. 5.6 Diagram of the intended line of transection

needles closest to the tumor, thus leaving coagulated liver parenchyma behind (Figs. 5.6 and 5.7). During transection, applying mild compression to the liver parenchyma helped the generated heat to seal vessels, thus contributing to a bloodless operative field.

Energy was either applied to the whole resection margin prior to cutting, or applied to partial sections dividing the liver parenchyma in a stepwise fashion. In order to coagulate deeper parts of the liver close to the IVC, the probe was introduced parallel to the IVC, and directed away from it. For tumors located adjacent to the liver hilum, dissection and ligation of the hilar structures were performed first, after which the probe was applied parallel and directed away from

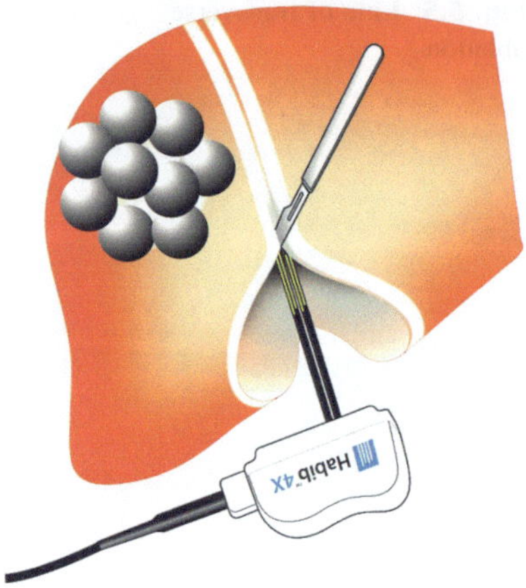

Fig. 5.7 Transection with a scalpel using the probe needles as a guide

the hilum. The power of the generator was set at 100 W for routine hepatic parenchymal coagulation. For sealing larger vessels such as hepatic veins, the power was lowered to 80 W. Decreasing the power paradoxically achieved a wider coagulation effect.

For deep tumors, the probe was introduced deep into the liver parenchyma guided by the surgeon's hand from below. After coagulation of the deepest part, the probe was withdrawn in a controlled manner to allow subsequent coagulation of the more superficial parts. The four needles of the probe were kept parallel to each other by lowering a push plate between them. This was necessary in order to prevent them from touching each other within the liver parenchyma, thus preventing short-circuiting.

Reference

1. Agrawal S, Belghiti J (2011) Oncologic resection for malignant tumors of the liver. Ann Surg 253:656–665

Ultrasonically Activated Device for Parenchymal Division During Open Liver Resection

6

Paolo Limongelli, Andrea Belli, Luigi Cioffi, Gianluca Russo, Alberto D'Agostino, Corrado Fantini and Giulio Belli

6.1 Introduction

Over the past decades, liver surgery has gained wide acceptance as a main therapeutic option for patients with both benign and malignant lesions. In the majority of series, morbidity and mortality improved significantly due to better patient selection and technical improvements [1]. Intraoperative blood loss during parenchymal transection was significantly reduced by either Glissonian approach or selective clamping and ligation of intrahepatic portal triads, together with use of low central venous pressure (CVP) maintenance during anesthesia [2]. Control of bleeding without causing hepatic ischemia still remains of utmost importance during performance of liver resection, since postoperative outcomes may be negatively influenced by intraoperative blood loss and intra- or perioperative transfusions [3]. The introduction of new technological devices has gained popularity among liver

---

Electronic Supplementary Material The online version of this article (doi:10.1007/978-88-470-2622-3_6) contains supplementary material which is available to authorized users.

P. Limongelli · A. Belli · L. Cioffi · G. Russo · A. D'Agostino · C. Fantini · G. Belli
Department of General and Hepato-Pancreato-Biliary Surgery, S.M. Loreto Nuovo Hospital, Naples, Italy
e-mail: limpao@libero.it
A. Belli
e-mail: belli.andrea@gmail.com

L. Cioffi
e-mail: luigi_cioffi@tin.it

G. Belli (✉)
Department of General and Hepato-Pancreato-Biliary Surgery, S. M. Loreto Nuovo Hospital
Via A. Vespucci, 80142 Naples, Italy
e-mail: chirurgia.loretonuovo@tin.it

I. Di Carlo (ed.), *Open, Laparoscopic and Robotic Hepatic Transection*,
DOI: 10.1007/978-88-470-2622-3_6, © Springer-Verlag Italia 2012

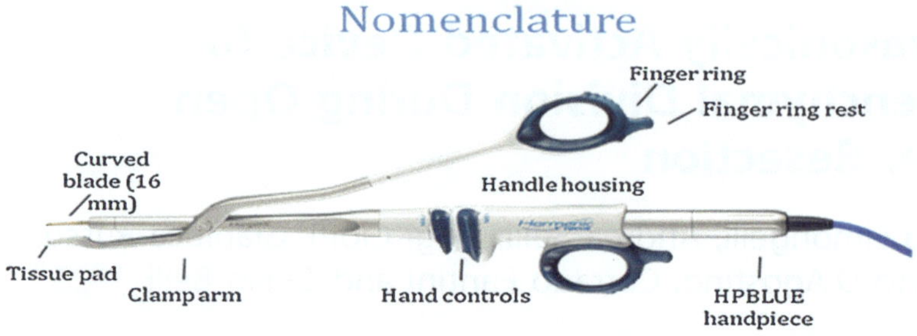

Fig. 6.1 Harmonic Focus® curved shears produce minimal lateral thermal spread (≤2 mm) near vital structures, enabling transection and sealing of vessels ≤5 mm as well as lymphatics

surgeons with the aim of improving safety of resection and reducing procedure-related complications such as bile leakage, hematoma, and infections.

In this chapter, we review the usefulness of the ultrasonic activated device (USAD) for dissection of liver parenchyma during open liver resection.

6.2 Device Description

The USAD (UltraSonic Harmonic Scalpel; Ethicon Endosurgery, Cincinnati, OH, USA) is composed of a generator emitting high-frequency alternating electric current with a foot switch; a handpiece containing an acoustic transducer triggering vibration caused by high-frequency electrical energy; and a single-use shears consisting of an upper anvil and an active lower blade which vibrates longitudinally at a harmonic frequency of 55,000 Hz. A blunt coagulation mode is used in order to attain good hemostasis, via slow cutting [4]. The tip of the vibrating blade has an excursion of 50,100 mm.

The lateral spread of the energy is estimated to be approximately 500 μm. The ultrasonic vibration energy acts by severing hydrogen bonds, which results in alteration of protein structures, intercellular dissection, and low-temperature vaporization of intra- and extracellular water, and hence the section of the tissue.

The local action of the instrument leads to the formation of a protein coagulum, which controls bleedings in vessels up to 3 mm in diameter and makes the tissue fragile enough to be dissected. The new Harmonic Focus (Fig. 6.1) is composed of a generator emitting high-frequency alternating electric current connected to a single-use handpiece containing an acoustic transducer triggering vibration caused by high-frequency electrical energy. The handpiece has a comfortable handle with two finger rings and power activating buttons. The clamp arm has a tissue pad and a curved blade specifically designed for fine and delicate dissection. The active blade vibrates longitudinally at a harmonic frequency of 55,000 Hz. The energy liberated as an ultrasound wave is applied directly to the tissue, thus accomplishing the triple effect of cavitation, coagulation, and cutting. The ultrasonic vibration energy acts by severing hydrogen bonds, which results in alteration of protein

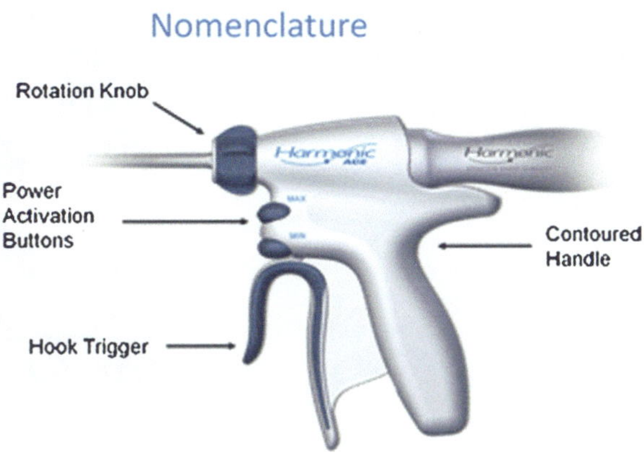

Fig. 6.2 Harmonic Ace® curved shears with jaw and curved blade enable precise dissection, sealing, and transection near vital structures and of vessels ≤5 mm and lymphatics

structures, intercellular dissection, and low-temperature vaporization of intra- and extracellular water, and hence the section of the tissue. The local action of the instrument leads to the formation of a protein coagulum and makes the tissue fragile enough to be dissected. The coagulating and sealing power of the new Harmonic Ace (Fig. 6.2) with an ergonomic open 23-cm-long handle allows efficient management of vessels and lymphatics of up to 5 mm. The lateral spread of the energy is estimated to be approximately 500 μm, thus minimizing lateral thermal tissue damage for safer dissection near vital structures.

6.3 Technique Description

Patient is placed in supine position with a pad. All operations are carried out under general anesthesia and controlled CVP maintained at <5 mmHg. Exploratory laparoscopy is conducted to assess the stage of the disease, and intraoperative ultrasound is performed to evaluate resectability. When resectability of the lesion(s) is ascertained, a right subcostal incision is performed and then extended in a J shape or to the left, if necessary.

Liver mobilization is accomplished according to planned liver resection; hepatogastric ligament is opened to inspect the Winslow foramen and to place a tourniquet around the hepatoduodenal ligament to perform a Pringle manoeuvre when necessary.

Hepatic arterial and portal vein branches are tied during formal hepatectomy, whilst hepatic veins are generally sutured with an extrahepatic approach using a vascular stapler. When resection regards one or more liver segment(s), the respective portal branches are suture-ligated.

Parenchymal transection starts under ultrasound guidance, incising the liver capsule with electrocautery to outline the surgical plane.

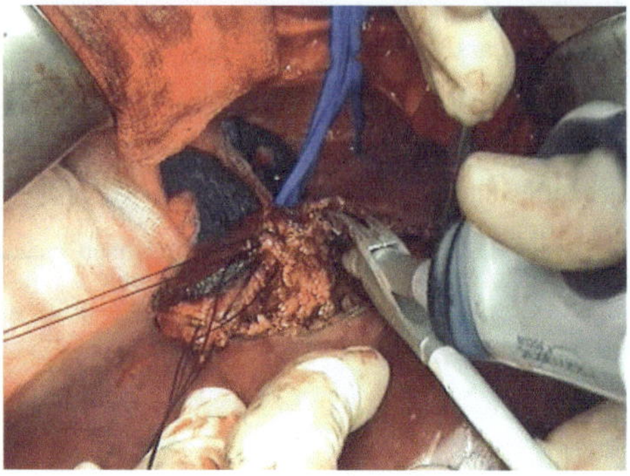

Fig. 6.3 Parenchymal transection under ultrasound guidance, using Harmonic Focus® curved shears

Subsegmental resections are performed without preventive vascular control. The USAD using medium energy at amplifier setting 3 and in blunt fashion is then employed to divide the liver tissue. Small bleedings may be managed by electrocautery, wet bipolar forceps, or USAD in flat coagulation mode. Larger vascular and biliary structures are exposed and electively tied and divided. Once resection is completed, the liver surface must be inspected for residual bleeding or bile leakage. Biologic fibrin glue (Tissucol; Baxter, Vienna, Austria) or a new hemostatic gel (Floseal; Baxter) can be applied on the raw liver surface.

The USAD, originally developed for laparoscopic general surgery, has been approved as a safe surgical instrument [5, 6]. The use of an ergonomic palmar handle harmonic scalpel and the clear view resulting from the very low smoke development, as well as a good coagulating effect, resulted very convincing in our laparoscopic liver resection experience [7].

In open surgery, this device can be used for blunt preparation, cutting, and coagulation, which are achieved by local thermal denaturation resulting from longitudinal vibration of the blade. Both thermal spreading and conduction have been shown to be significantly lower when compared with electrocoagulation and laser [8]. As during laparoscopic liver surgery [14], we approach the cut surface of the liver from up to down, layer by layer [9–11]. Once the liver capsule is marked by electrocautery, the ultrasonic blades are closed progressively in blunt fashion up to 2–3 cm depth circumferentially along the resection plan (Fig. 6.3). This allows safe and effective transection, also in a cirrhotic liver. When liver dissection continues deeply in the liver, the USAD has to be applied for longer time but in flat coagulation mode to control small bleedings. In close proximity to large venous branches, as occurs during major hepatic resections, USAD may damage the vessel wall, causing tedious bleeding that can disturb further steps of the procedure [12]. We perform the Pringle maneuver only in selected cases, since this maneuver has been previously debated, especially in cirrhotic patients [7]. Employment of USAD may help surgeons avoid this maneuver thanks to its hemostatic effect during parenchymal transaction, even in cirrhotic liver. It has also been reported in association with a plain and brownish cut surface of the liver, partly explaining why biliary leaks or persistent bleeding can easily be detected and treated [13].

Use of an argon beam coagulator or fibrin glue at the end of parenchyma transection may improve sealing of the raw liver surface and ensure hemostasis and biliostasis.

In a retrospective study, the USAD was found to be effective and superior to ultrasonic aspirator in reducing blood loss and shortening the time of the operation, suggesting its employment during limited liver resections with cirrhosis or chronic hepatitis [14]. Whrightson et al. reported that concomitant utilization of USAD and vascular stapler provides relatively bloodless dissection only on the surface of the liver, but carries a high rate of biliary leakage [15] due to incomplete sealing of all bile ducts. The authors suggest combined use of new technologies to reduce the need for blood transfusion and Pringle maneuver and the associated risk of postoperative liver dysfunction. In our opinion, use of new technological devices may encourage general surgeons to perform minor liver resections with fair feasibility and safety, and popularize liver surgery as an optimal therapeutic choice in management of liver tumors (such as small synchronous colorectal liver metastases), instead of alternative ablative procedures.

In conclusion, although there is a lack of data based on well-conducted controlled studies and further studies on a greater number of patients are needed, according to our experience, utilization of USAD may help to minimize blood loss during liver resection regardless of the condition of the liver, even in case of cirrhosis.

References

1. Weber JC, Navarra G, Jiao LR (2002) New technique for liver resection using heat coagulative necrosis. Ann Surg 236(5):560–563
2. Moug SJ, Smith D, Leen E, Angerson WJ, Horgan PG (2007) Selective continuous vascular occlusion and perioperative fluid restriction in partial hepatectomy. Outcomes in 101 consecutive patients. Eur J Surg Oncol 33(8):1036–1041
3. de Boer MT, Molenaar IQ, Porte RJ (2007) Impact of blood loss on outcome after liver resection. Dig Surg 24(4):259–264
4. Fritze F, Lorenz D (2001) The application of the ultrasoni scalpel in liver surgery. In: Kö ckerling F, Scwartz SI (eds) Liver surgery. Operative techniques and avoidance of complications. J.A. Barth, Heidelberg, pp 77–81
5. Cugat E, Hoyuela C, Rodriguez-Santiago JM, Marco C (1999) Laparoscopic resection of benign gastric tumors. J Laparoendosc Adv Surg Tech A 9:63–67
6. Jackman SV, Cadeddu JA, Chen RN, Micali S, Bishoff JT, Lee BR, Moore RG, Kavoussi LR (1998) Utility of the harmonic scalpel for laparoscopic partial nephrectomy. J Endourol 12:441–444
7. Belli G, Fantini C, D'Agostino A, Belli A, Cioffi L, Russolillo N (2006) Laparoscopic left lateral lobectomy: a safer and faster technique. J Hepatobiliary Pancreas Surg 13:149–154
8. Geller DA, Tsung A, Maheshwari V, Rutstein LA, Fung JJ, Marsh W (2005) Hepatic resection in 170 patients using salinecooled radiofrequency coagulation. HPB 7:208–213
9. Belli G, D'Agostino A, Fantini C, Cioffi L, Belli A, Limongelli P, Russo G (2009) Surgical treatment of giant liver hemangiomas by enucleation using an ultrasonically activated device (USAD). Hepatogastroenterology 56(89):236–239

10. Belli G, Fantini C, D'Agostino A, Cioffi L, Langella S, Russolillo N, Belli A (2007) Laparoscopic versus open liver resection for hepatocellular carcinoma in patients with histologically proven cirrhosis: short- and middle-term results. Surg Endosc 21(11):2004–2011
11. Belli G, D'Agostino A, Ciciliano F, Fantini C, Russolillo N, Belli A (2002) Liver resection for hepatic metastases: 15 years of experience. J Hepatobiliary Pancreat Surg 9(5):607–613
12. Sugo H, Matsumoto K, Kojima K, Fukasawa M, Beppu T (2005) Role of ultrasonically activated scalpel in hepatic resection: a comparison with conventional blunt dissection. Hepatogastroenterology 52:173–175
13. Schmidbauer S, Hallfeldt KK, Sitzmann G, Kantelhardt T, Trupka A (2002) Experience with ultrasound scissors and blades (UltraCision) in open and laparoscopic liver resection. Ann Surg 235:27–30
14. Ouchi K, Mikuni J, Sugawara T, Ono H, Fujiya T, Kamiyama Y, Kakugawa Y, Yamanami H, Nakagawa K (2000) Hepatectomyusing an ultrasonically activated scalpel for hepatocellular carcinoma. Dig Surg 17:138–142
15. Whrightson WR, Edward MJ, McMasters KM (2000) The role of the ultrasonically activated shears and vascular cutting stapler in hepatic resection. Am Surg 66:1037–1040

Open Hepatic Transection Using Water-Jet Dissector

7

Kerstin Huepgens, Denis Ehrl and Horst-Guenter Rau

7.1 Principles of Dissection

The liver consists of a three-dimensional network of afferent and efferent duct and vessel systems. Because of the higher content of collagen and elastin, these duct and vessel systems differ essentially in their structure and resistance from the liver parenchyma.

Due to these physical properties, it is possible to release and dissect the duct and vessel systems mechanically from the liver parenchyma [1].

Dissection techniques which take advantage of these anatomic conditions are called selective; these include blunt dissection, the CUSA technique, and water-jet dissection.

The nonselective dissection techniques are the scalpel, scissor, linear stapler, high-frequency coagulation, the UltraCision®, and the laser technique. These techniques do not discriminate between duct structures and parenchyma.

Electronic Supplementary Material The online version of this article (doi:10.1007/978-88-470-2622-3_7) contains supplementary material which is available to authorized users.

K. Huepgens (✉) · D. Ehrl · H.-G. Rau
Surgical Department of Visceral and Thoracic Surgery, Amper Klinikum Dachau, Krankenhaussstrasse 15, 85221 Dachau, Germany
e-mail: kerstin.huepgens@amperkliniken.de

D. Ehrl
e-mail: denis.ehrl@amperkliniken.de

H.-G. Rau
e-mail: Gabriele.Stichlmayr@amperkliniken.de

I. Di Carlo (ed.), *Open, Laparoscopic and Robotic Hepatic Transection*,
DOI: 10.1007/978-88-470-2622-3_7, © Springer-Verlag Italia 2012

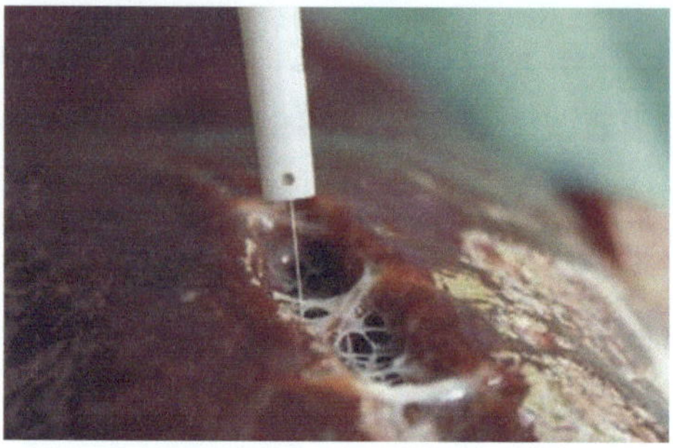

Fig. 7.1 Liver resection with water-jet dissector

Using the water-jet dissector, the blood vessels and bile ducts are prepared and washed free of surrounding tissue with the help of precisely adjusted water pressure (Fig. 7.1). The water-jet dissector acts thereby like an intelligent knife. Depending on their size, the blood vessels and bile ducts can then be either coagulated or selectively treated using a ligature/clip.

The aims of all these devices are reduction of intraoperative blood loss, avoidance of parenchymal trauma, and reduction of Pringle rate and operation time.

7.2 Device Description

Cutting with a high-pressure water jet was a development that was primarily used as an industrial technique. At pressure levels of about 20,000 bar, a water jet reaches supersonic speed at the tip of the nozzle, which enables effortless cutting of wood and even steel plates without development of heat [1].

For application in surgery, the nozzle tip and pressure parameters had to be adjusted to the structural properties of parenchymal organs. The first development was made by Papachristou and Bengmark [2, 3], who implemented the technology in experimental and clinical investigations. Simultaneously, the working group of Rau et al. refined this technique based on the results of in vitro and in vivo trials, and after improvement introduced it into clinical routine liver surgery in 1990. In experimental examinations, we found that pressure of 30–40 bar and nozzle diameter of 0.1 mm is very effective to dissect normal liver tissue. In case of cirrhotic liver parenchyma, the pressure needed for dissection is 10 bar higher. Above these parameters, the quality of dissection becomes worse and the rate of vessel injuries, especially of the hepatic veins, increases, with corresponding higher blood loss [4].

Despite the positive clinical experiences, it took another 6 years until the first commercial devices were available.

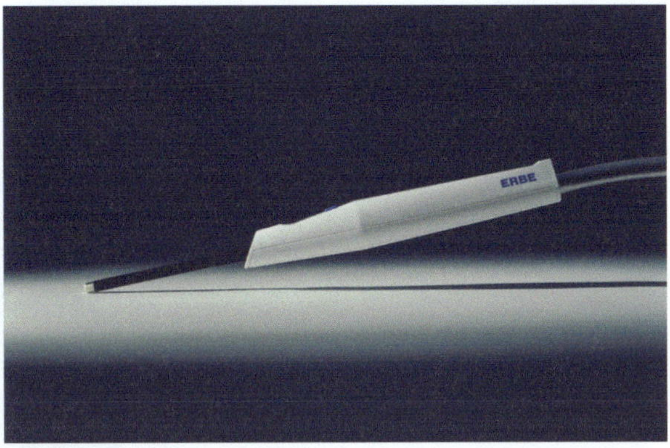

Fig. 7.2 Handpiece (Erbe Medizinmechanik GmbH, Tuebingen, Germany)

7.3 Technique Description

In open surgery, the water-jet dissector is used with nozzle diameter of 0.1 mm and pressure of 30–40 bar (Fig. 7.2).

Up to now, we have used six different types of water-jet dissectors which were continuously improved regarding handpieces and practicability. The latest model is shown in Fig. 7.3.

As the jet liquid we use physiological sodium solution. For hemihepatectomy, we usually need about 400 ml jet solution.

The standard procedure in open surgery starts with preparation of hilar vessels and hepatic veins prior to parenchyma dissection. The right hemiliver is completely mobilized from the diaphragm. After this, we use intraoperative ultrasound to detect the localization of the tumor and its proximity to the vessels.

After this, the resection line is defined. During dissection we practice well-organized work-sharing between dissection, clipping of dissected vessels, and cutting them between the clips.

The advantage of the water-jet dissector is the closing of the thin-walled veins in the depth of the parenchyma and the avoidance of difficult bleedings. In contrast, the CUSA, LigaSure, or bipolar scissors are less efficient at depth. They can be effectively used in the surface area of the liver, because only here can they achieve good hemostasis.

Since 2010, we have used a handpiece with additional application of high-frequency current. With this method, it is possible to coagulate small vessels and bile ducts instead of clipping. As a result, the operation time is again reduced significantly.

Use of the handpiece with high-frequency current showed no increase in bile duct leaks in comparison with the handpiece without high-frequency current.

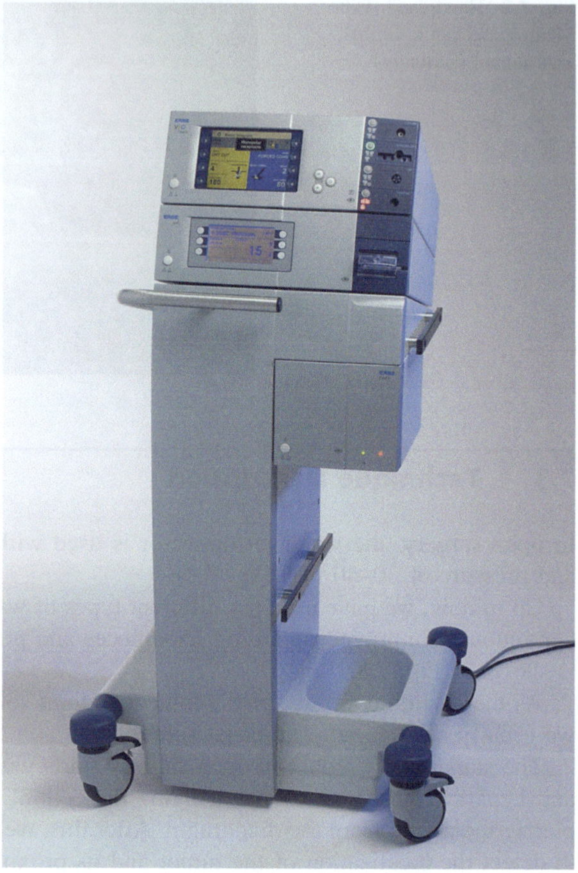

Fig. 7.3 Water jet (Erbe Elektromedizin GmbH, Tuebingen, Germany)

7.4 Complications and Results

In the beginning, the water-jet dissection technique was assessed very critically, especially in oncological resection. It was feared that the water jet might penetrate liver tissue without control, so that it would contact the tumor and tumor cells could be spread into the operating field. In this way, the local recurrence rate might increase and overall survival might decrease.

However, analysis of overall survival following resection of liver metastases and hepatocellular carcinoma showed that the dissection technique has no influence on long-term survival. In a comparative clinical study between different dissection techniques (water jet, CUSA, and blunt dissection) in 591 patients who underwent liver resection, no significant differences were found between Kaplan–Meier survival curves, even in cases of extended liver resections [5, 6].

Table 7.1 Development of operation parameters in liver resection using the water jet over the course of 20 years

	1991–1996	1997–2002	2003–2007	2008–2011
n	96	120	137	178
Pringle rate (%)	46	48	6	0.6
Operating time (min)	214	294	181	170
Blood loss (ml)	1442.6	1337.9	523.7	492.1
EC per patient	1.86	0.71	0.46	0.44

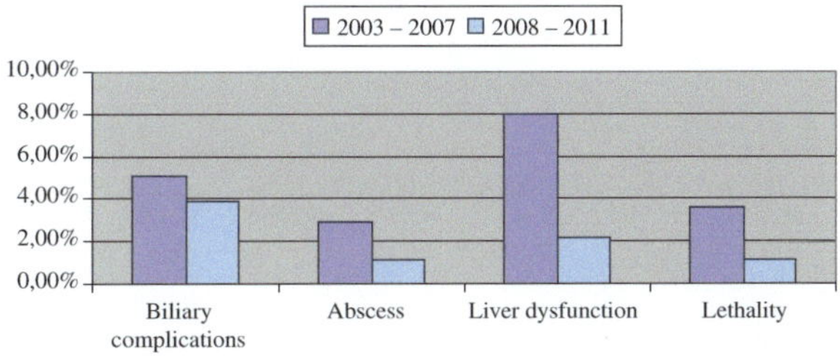

Fig. 7.4 Postoperative complications after liver resection using the water jet

With the water-jet dissection technique, it is possible to reduce the Pringle rate, operating time, blood loss, and postoperative complications after liver resection (Table 7.1; Fig. 7.4).

In the last 9 years, in over 90 % of liver resections and even in extended liver resections (two segments and more) we did not perform a Pringle manoeuvre, without an increase of blood loss (Table 7.1).

Based on these positive results of using the water-jet dissector, we implemented this technique as our standard dissection procedure in open and laparoscopic liver surgery.

References

1. Rau HG, Schauer R, Pickelmann S, Meyer BCM, Angele MK, Zimmermann A, Meimarakis G, Heizmann O, Schildberg FW (2001) Dissektionstechniken in der Leberchirurgie. Chirurg 73:105–112
2. Bengmark S (1987) Leberchirurgie. Chir Gastroenterol 3:5–11
3. Papachristou DN, Barters R (1982) Resection of the liver with a water jet. Br J Surg 69:93–94
4. Rau HG, Arnold H, Schildberg FW (1990) Schneiden mit dem Wasser-Strahl (Jet-Cutting)– eine Alternative zum Ultraschallaspirator? Chirurg 61:735–738

5. Rau HG, Wichmann M, Schinkel S, Buttler E, Pickelmann S, Schauer R (2001) Surgical techniques in hepatic resections: ultrasonic aspirator versus jet cutter–a prospective randomized clinical trial. Zentralbl Chir 126:586–590
6. Rau HG, Zimmermann A, Wardemann C, Schildberg FW (2003) Standards of surgical techniques in liver metastases. Chir Gastroenterol 19:333–339

Open Hepatic Transection Using Kelly Clamp

8

Takuya Hashimoto, Norihiro Kokudo and Masatoshi Makuuchi

8.1 Introduction

Minimization of blood loss during hepatic resection still remains a major concern for liver surgeons. Thus, surgical techniques and devices have been developed to achieve control of blood loss [1], although the safety of hepatic resection itself has already been established [2]. The method used for liver transection has been considered to be the most critical factor influencing intraoperative blood loss.

Hepatic parenchyma may be transected by conventional digitoclasia (finger fracture [3]), clamp-crushing [4] or with instrument-based techniques (ultrasonic, water-jet dissector, saline-linked radiofrequency coagulator, and a vessel sealing system). The procedure used depends solely on surgeon training or preference rather than objective data.

Electronic Supplementary Material The online version of this article (doi: 10.1007/978-88-470-2622-3_8) contains supplementary material which is available to authorized users.

T. Hashimoto · M. Makuuchi (✉)
Department of Hepato-Biliary-Pancreatic Surgery,
Japanese Red Cross Medical Center, Shibuya-ku, Tokyo, Japan
e-mail: masatoshi.makuuchi@gmail.com

T. Hashimoto
e-mail: Thashimo-tky@umin.ac.jp

N. Kokudo
Department of Hepato-Biliary-Pancreatic Surgery, Department of Artificial Organ and Transplantation, Graduate School of Medicine, University of Tokyo, Bunkyo-ku, Tokyo, Japan
e-mail: KOKUDO-2SU@h.u-tokyo.ac.jp

I. Di Carlo (ed.), *Open, Laparoscopic and Robotic Hepatic Transection*,
DOI: 10.1007/978-88-470-2622-3_8,

We prefer to use the conventional Kelly clamp method, because this method is safe, quick, and inexpensive. We have previously conducted randomized controlled studies to prove the usefulness of using various types of equipment for liver resection, but advantages of these devices were not proven over conventional techniques [5–9]. In this chapter, we present keys to successful performance of the "Kelly clamp method".

8.2 Device Description

For the Kelly clamp method, no special device is required except for forceps as used in usual surgery. Forceps of adequate size and shape to clamp a small amount of liver parenchyma is selected according to the stiffness of the liver and the situation of the resection.

In the past, we have used pediatric Kelly forceps for clamping [4], but today, we prefer to use a larger-size Péan forceps (Rochester Péan 18 cm, 32-01125; Leibinger, Germany; Fig. 8.1). The size seems suitable for the various conditions of liver parenchyma. The tip of this tool is curved and not sharply pointed, and the shape is useful in seeking and exposing the varied vessels in the liver parenchyma without unnecessary bleeding or injury.

8.3 Technique Description

Keys to the "Kelly clamp method" are:

1. Crushing of a certain amount of liver parenchyma using a Péan forceps
2. Aspiration of the crushed tissues using an aspirator
3. Ligation and division of the remaining structures including vessels and bile ducts

The resection line at the surface of the liver is marked by electrocautery. After the blood flow of the liver is totally or selectively occluded at the hepatic hilum, division of the hepatic parenchyma is commenced.

At the first stage of parenchymal division, a Péan forceps with opened tips is penetrated vertically along the coagulated resection line. The width of the opened tips should be 5 to 10 mm (Fig. 8.2). Then, the forceps is gently controlled to clamp two or three times to crush the liver parenchyma. This motion is repeated horizontally along the resection planes to the targeted vessels (Fig. 8.3). Crushed liver parenchyma should remain on both sides of the planes. The assistants should then remove these tissues and blood using an aspirator suction tube, leaving the small vessels bridging between the divided planes (Fig. 8.4). Forceps is inserted from under these bridging tissues by the operator, the assistant ligates the vessels using 3-0 or 4-0 silk at the remaining side of the liver, and the operator divides these structures by scissors (Figs. 8.5 and 8.6), and for thick portal pedicle of more than 3 mm, 2-0 silk is used with or without 3-0 Ti-Cron transfixion suture. The width of the clamp should be

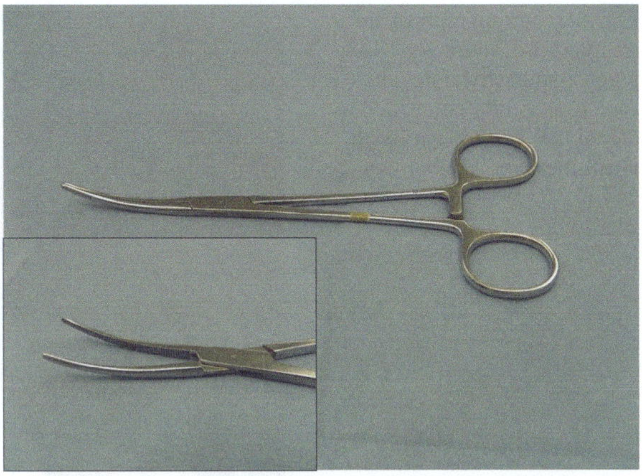

Fig. 8.1 Photograph of Péan forceps (Rochester Péan 18 cm, 32-01125; Leibinger, Germany). The tip is curved and not sharply pointed

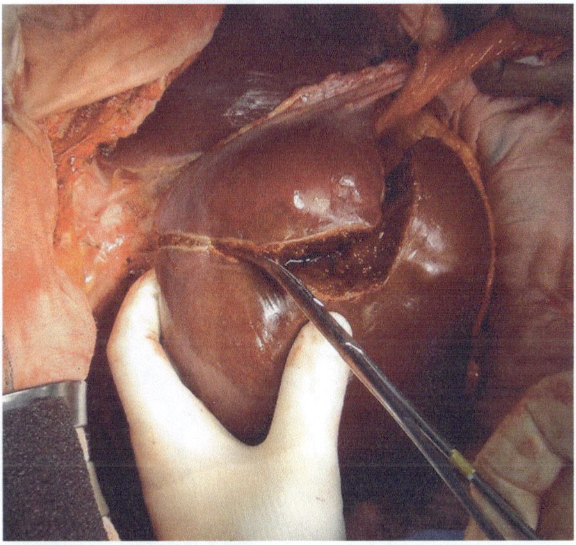

Fig. 8.2 Photograph of the standard procedure for parenchymal division. A Péan forceps with opened tips is penetrated vertically along the coagulated resection line in extended right hepatectomy

adjusted according to the condition of the liver. When the liver is cirrhotic and hard, the width of the opened tips of the forceps should be narrow to avoid tearing the vessels to be ligated. Bleeding from the resection plane is more remarkable until the depth of the resection reaches about 1 cm from the surface of the liver, compared with when dividing the deeper part of the liver. Sufficient operative view at the deeper part of the liver is obtained by dividing the liver parenchyma also in the antero-posterior direction and widening the surgical area. Basic procedures for division of the deeper part of the liver are the same as described above.

The obstacles during liver division are the portal pedicles and hepatic veins. The operator has to decide which vessels should be divided or preserved according to the type of the scheduled operation. In anatomical resection, tumor bearing

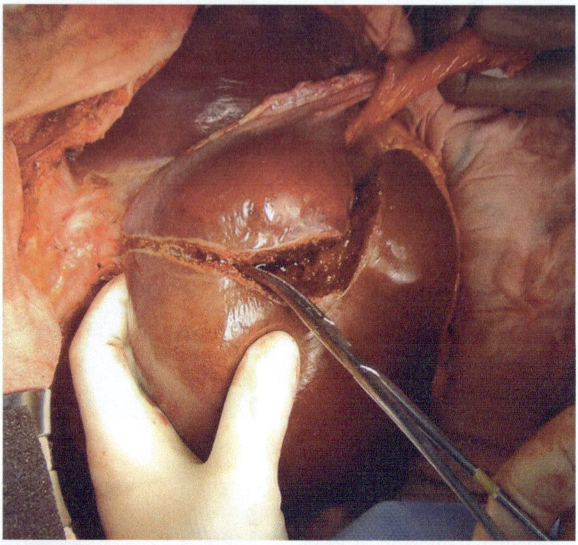

Fig. 8.3 Photograph of the standard procedure for parenchymal division. The forceps is gently controlled to clamp two or three times to crush the liver parenchyma

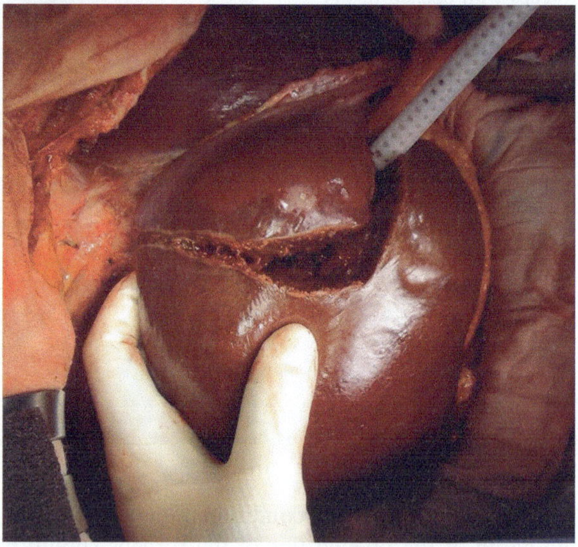

Fig. 8.4 Photograph of the standard procedure for parenchymal division. After removal of the crushed parenchymal tissues and blood using an aspirator suction tube by the assistants, the small vessels are left bridging the divided planes

portal pedicles is ligated and divided at the point where the size of these vessels is relatively thick. Under ultrasonic guidance, the resection plane of the target portal pedicle can be reached. The portal pedicle with surrounding liver parenchyma is clamped just enough to expose the portal pedicle. Then, the portal pedicle is exposed longitudinally about 5 mm to 1 cm in length. When there are tiny branches ramifying near the ligation point, these branches should be meticulously exposed, ligated, and divided before division of the main portal pedicle. The tip of the forceps should not be penetrated deeply, because occasionally there is a hepatic

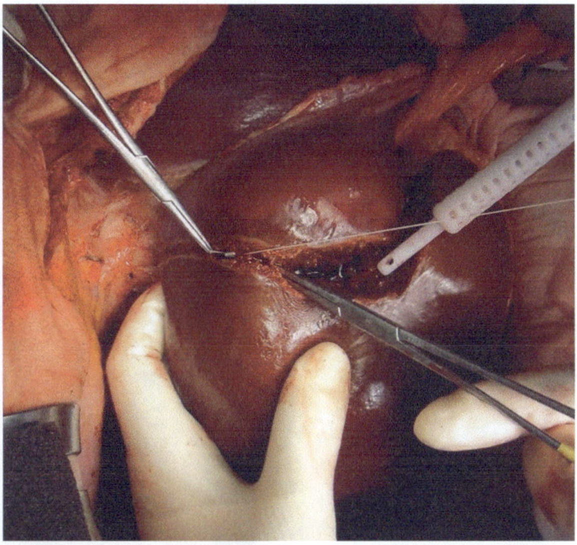

Fig. 8.5 Photograph of the standard procedure for parenchymal division. Forceps is inserted from under the bridging tissues by the operator, and the operator catches the silk with the forceps

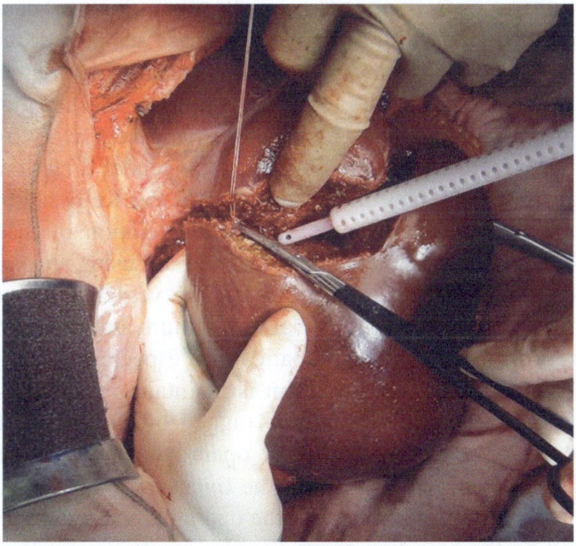

Fig. 8.6 Photograph of the standard procedure for parenchymal division. After the vessels at the remaining side of the liver are ligated by the assistant, the operator divides these structures by scissors

vein running behind the target portal pedicle. The portal pedicle with a certain diameter should then be doubly ligated with transfixing suture and divided.

In anatomical resection, the landmark hepatic veins should be preserved and exposed on the raw surface of the liver. A part of the hepatic vein is exposed under guidance of ultrasonography. Along this exposed vein, the liver parenchyma in front of the hepatic vein is clamped and widely divided. A small part of the hepatic venous wall is gently peeled off from the liver parenchyma using the tip of the

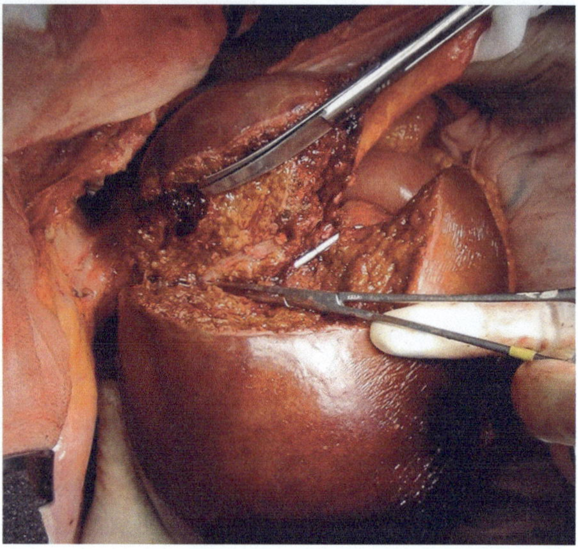

Fig. 8.7 Photograph of the exposure of the hepatic vein. The middle hepatic vein is widely exposed. The small tributaries are carefully exposed, ligated, and divided

forceps or scissors. The small tributaries are carefully exposed, ligated, and divided (Fig. 8.7). The tiny tributaries are pulled out from the parenchyma using De Bakey or Cooley pincettes, and finally, semicircumference of the hepatic vein is exposed. To avoid tearing the forks of the hepatic venous tributaries, a suction tube is moved gently along the hepatic vein away from the inferior vena cava, in other words, from the cranial to the caudal direction.

Assistants play important roles in the Kelly clamp method. The main roles of the assistants are quick and certain ligation of the vessels, maintenance of the operative field, and keeping the field dry using an aspirator. The first assistant must quickly ligate even the tiniest of the vessels without tearing or pulling them out from the thicker venous wall. Maximum attention should be paid to ligation of the tiny tributaries of the hepatic vein, especially when the hepatic vein is exposed. Another role of the assistant is maintaining a good surgical view by countertraction. One resection plane is tugged by the assistant and another is held by the operator. Securing sufficient operative view will become more difficult as you proceed deeper away from the liver surface. Therefore, assistants are required to work closely together with the operator, and secure the operative view by carefully lifting the resection plane thereby maintaining adequate angle. Aspiration by the second assistant is equally important. The assistant should aspirate the crushed tissues and/or blood at all times from the opposite side of the proceeding hepatic parenchymal division during the procedure. When aspirating the front of the dividing plane, the tip of the aspirator should be moved gently, smoothly skimming the crushed parenchymal tissues and/or blood. Excessive pressure should not be applied at the tip of the aspirator to avoid unnecessary injury.

The Kelly clamp method (clamp-crushing method) is a simple and certain method for hepatic parenchymal division, and mastering the method would lead to safer liver surgery.

References

1. Poon RT (2007) Current techniques of liver transection. HPB (Oxford) 9:166–173
2. Imamura H, Seyama Y, Kokudo N, et al. (2003) One thousand fifty-six hepatectomies without mortality in 8 years. Arch Surg 138:1198–1206 (discussion 1206)
3. Lin TY (1974) A simplified technique for hepatic resection: the crush method. Ann Surg 180:285–290
4. Makuuchi M, Hasegawa H, Yamazaki S (1985) Ultrasonically guided subsegmentectomy. Surg Gynecol Obstet 161:346–350
5. Takayama T, Makuuchi M, Kubota K et al. (2001) Randomized comparison of ultrasonic vs. clamp resection of the liver. Arch Surg 136:922–928
6. Arita J, Hasegawa K, Kokudo N et al. (2005) Randomized clinical trial of the effect of a saline-linked radiofrequency coagulator on blood loss during hepatic resection. Br J Surg 92:954–959
7. Seyama Y, Makuuchi M, Takayama T et al. (2005) Can a small ultrasonic dissector equipped for electrocautery improve the results of hepatic resection? Hepatogastroenterology 52:1845–1848
8. Ikeda M, Hasegawa K, Sano K et al. (2009) The vessel sealing system (LigaSure) in hepatic resection: a randomized controlled trial. Ann Surg 250:199–203
9. Saiura A, Yamamoto J, Koga R et al. (2006) Usefulness of LigaSure for liver resection: analysis by randomized clinical trial. Am J Surg 192:41–45

9 Open Hepatic Transection Using LigaSure

Akio Saiura and Junji Yamamoto

9.1 Introduction

The clamp-crush (CC) technique is considered the current standard technique for liver transection [1]. There are two steps in conventional liver transection using the CC technique; the first is to expose the vessels including the hepatic vein and Glisson's sheath, and the second is to ligate or ablate the residual tissues by electric cautery. LigaSure™ tissue fusion, like LigaSure™ vessel sealing (Valleylab, Boulder, CO), uses the body's own collagen and elastin to create a permanent fusion zone. In a randomized clinical trial, use of the LigaSure™ system reduced operation time and blood loss in patients undergoing various surgical procedures including gynecological, colorectal, urological, and general surgery [2–4]. When used in liver transection, LigaSure™ can seal and cut vessels faster than manual ligation and is more consistent and reliable than conventional electric cautery. We previously reported that use of a prototype LigaSure™ system plus CC technique during liver resection allowed rapid and safe division of liver parenchyma [5].

Electronic Supplementary Material The online version of this article (doi:10.1007/978-88-470-2622-3_9) contains supplementary material which is available to authorized users.

A. Saiura (✉)
Department of Gastroenterological Surgery, Cancer Institute Ariake Hospital, Japanese Foundation for Cancer Research, Koto-ku, Tokyo, Japan
e-mail: saiura-tky@umin.ac.jp

I. Di Carlo (ed.), *Open, Laparoscopic and Robotic Hepatic Transection*,
DOI: 10.1007/978-88-470-2622-3_9,

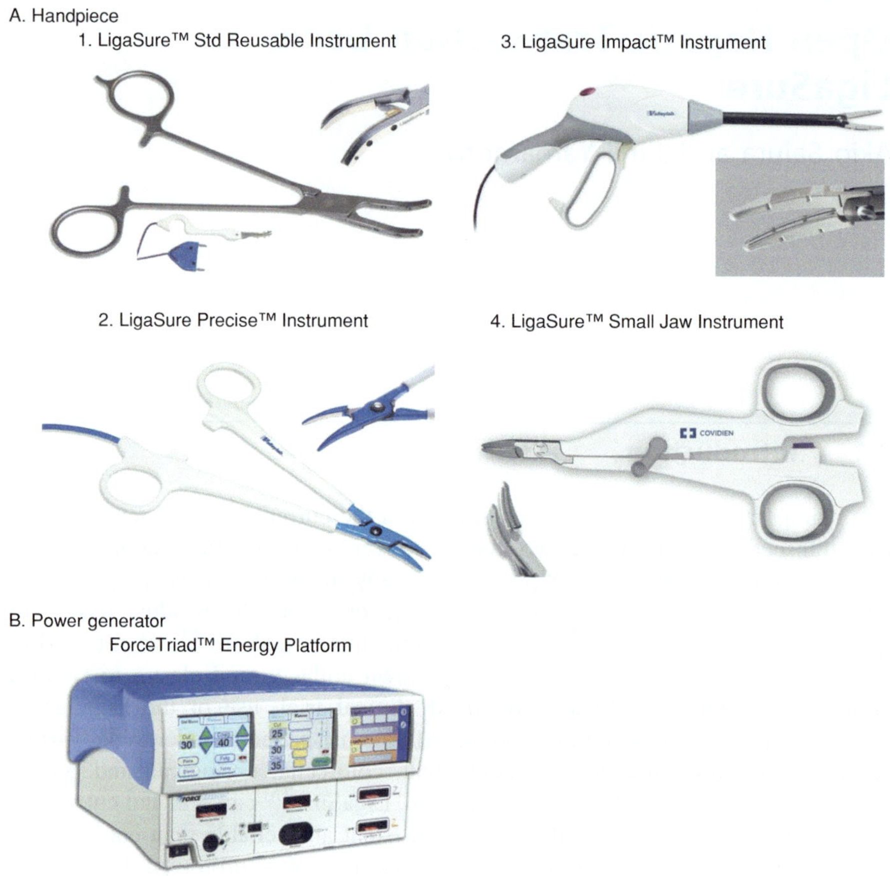

Fig. 9.1 Various types of handpiece and power generator of LigaSure™ system

LigaSure™ has the best synergy with the CC technique [6]. The LigaSure™ system, including the equipment such as the handpiece and energy platform, has been improved, and we can transect liver parenchyma more easily and quickly with the new system [7].

9.2 Device Description

LigaSure™ is basically a bipolar electric cautery. The LigaSure™ system is made up of an energy platform and handpiece. LigaSure™ tissue fusion, like LigaSure™ vessel sealing, uses the body's own collagen and elastin to create a permanent fusion zone. This technology can fuse vessels as large as 7 mm, lymphatics, and tissue bundles quickly and safely. Since the debut of LigaSure™ in 1998, the energy platform and handpiece of the LigaSure™ vessel sealing

Table 9.1 Comparison of LigaSure™ handpieces

Type of handpiece	Standard (Std™)	Precise™	Impact™	Small Jaw™
Debut year	2000	2001	2009	2011
Function	Sealer	Sealer	Sealer/divider	Sealer/divider
Size	Medium	Small	Large	Small
Shape of tip	Angular	Round	Round	Round
Speed	Medium	Medium	Fast	Fast: 2–4 s
Sealing quality	△	○	○	◎
Thin tissue	×	○	×	◎
Thick tissue	○	×	◎	○
Reuse	Reusable	Disposable	Disposable	Disposable
Cost	Low	Medium	High	High

system have both been updated and improved. LigaSure™ tissue fusion now uses the ForceTriad™ energy platform, which is controlled by TissueFect™ sensing technology and has faster fusion cycles, more flexible fusion zones, and less desiccation than the original LigaSure™ generator. The handpiece has also been improved in shape and function (Fig. 9.1). Various types of handpieces are now available, depending on surgeon preference. The characteristics of the four types of LigaSure™ handpieces are described in Table 9.1. Handpiece selection is most important for achieving the maximum potential of the system. LigaSure Impact™ and LigaSure™ Small Jaw have a divider to seal and cut the tissue synchronously. The shape of the tip is also very important to avoid traumatic injury of tiny vessels after crushing liver parenchyma. In combination with CC technique using Kelly forceps, the small, round tip is the best. LigaSure™ Small Jaw, which is the newest handpiece, has the fastest tissue fusion with the newest energy platform (ForceTriad™). Moreover, fusion of small, thin vessels, such as branches of the hepatic vein, by the round, small tip of the LigaSure™ Small Jaw is reliable. Overall, the LigaSure™ Small Jaw has the best synergy with the original CC technique.

9.3 Technical Description

After laparotomy, the whole liver was examined by intraoperative ultrasonography. Liver transection was performed using CC technique and an intermittent Pringle maneuver with periods of 15 min of clamping and 5 min of unclamping. In our original study of the prototype LigaSure™ system, we used the medium-sized handpiece (LigaSure™ Std) with the original power platform, and liver transection was accomplished in three steps [5] (Fig. 9.2). First, the liver parenchyma was

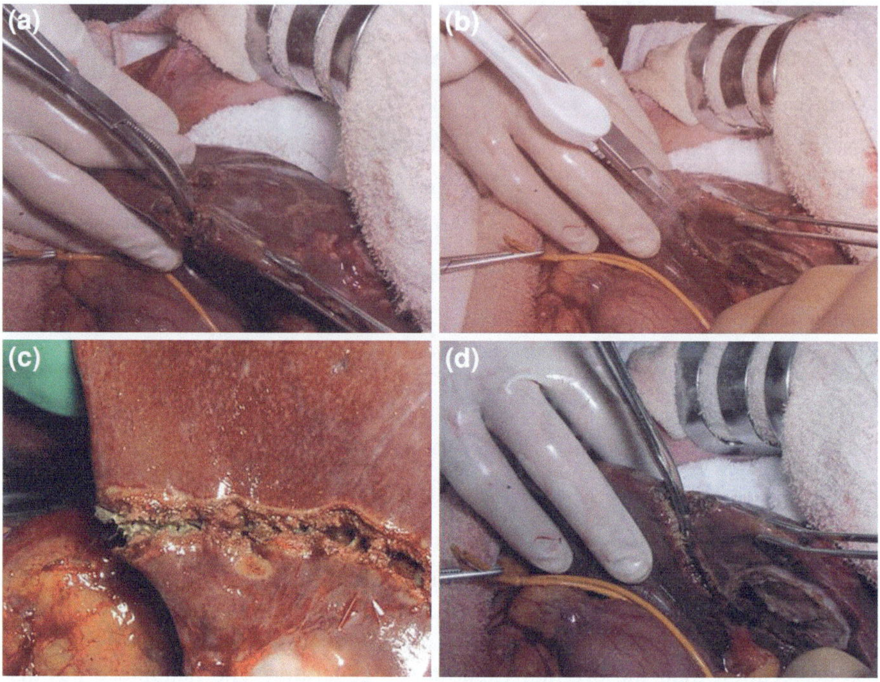

Fig. 9.2 Procedure of liver transection using LigaSure™ Std reusable instrument

crushed using Kelly forceps (Fig. 9.2a) and then aspirated, revealing the residual vessels or Glisson's sheaths. Second, the residual tissue was sealed using the LigaSure™ (Fig. 9.2b, c) at power level 2. Glisson's sheaths or hepatic veins of greater than 3 mm diameter were ligated with 4-0 Vicryl (Ethicon, Somerville, NJ) (Fig. 9.3). Finally, the center of the sealed zone was divided with scissors (Fig. 9.2d), and electric cautery was used to seal the remaining tissue. No clips were used.

LigaSure Precise™ is a finer handpiece that can create fusion of thin and small vessels; however, the sealing zone is too narrow to cut the center with scissors precisely. Thus, in a randomized controlled trial [6] using this handpiece, the transection speed was similar to the original CC technique. LigaSure Impact™ and LigaSure™ Small Jaw are second-generation handpieces with the new function of divider plus inner cutter. With this new function, vessels can be cut and divided in a single step, saving time and reducing blood loss. LigaSure™ Small Jaw is the most recent handpiece developed and the best handpiece currently available. The small and smooth shape of the tip is good for introducing into the narrow space after crushing the liver parenchyma with Kelly forceps. LigaSure™ Small Jaw can crush soft liver parenchyma; however, the result is not as good as crushing by Kelly forceps, especially when dealing with hard, cirrhotic liver parenchyma.

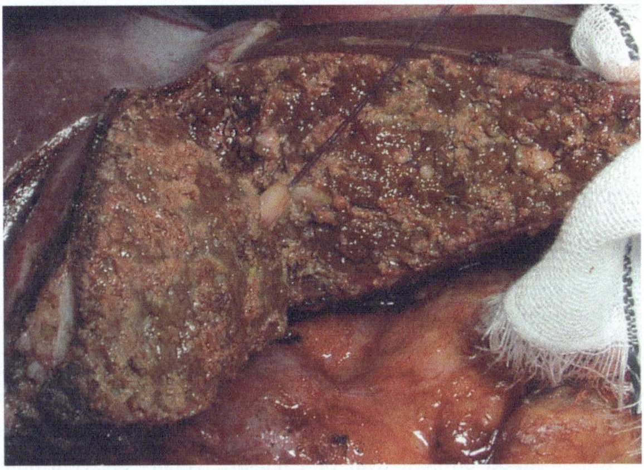

Fig. 9.3 Raw surface of liver transection and ligated Glisson's sheath of segment 3

9.4 Complication and Results

LigaSure™ can seal vessels up to 7 mm in diameter. In contrast to the high reliability of sealing medium-sized vessels, there were two weaknesses that needed to be improved in the prototype LigaSure™ (LigaSure™ Std). One was the high frequency of sealing errors with thin vessels such as branches of the hepatic vein. The other was the sealing speed. These limitations have been improved by the enhancement of the handpiece and the energy platform.

In contrast to its vessel fusion ability, the reliability of LigaSure™ in sealing bile ducts is unclear. Glisson's sheath includes bile ducts; therefore, a thick Glisson's sheath larger than 3 mm should be ligated. In our previous report, the incidence of postoperative bile leakage was similar with LigaSure™ compared with the original CC technique. There are no major vessels in the liver surface (<1 cm from the surface) or in the plane of the portal fissure. LigaSure™ can transect such areas without ligation. In our randomized trial using LigaSure™, the average number of ligations during liver transection was only six, which was significantly fewer than the number used during the original CC technique [5].

Exposing the major hepatic vein is an important anatomical procedure in liver resection. Controlling bleeding from the small hepatic vein branches is the main technique in this procedure. LigaSure™ Small Jaw can seal such thin hepatic vein branches without injury. This helps to expose the hepatic vein easily and safely.

Crushing the parenchyma and exposing the vessels using Kelly forceps is the most important step, as in the original CC technique. Incomplete crushing may result in incomplete sealing of vessels ("half seal"), which may cause bleeding or postoperative bile leakage.

The morbidity of liver resection in patients with cirrhosis of the liver is higher [8]. Crushing the hard liver parenchyma and exposing the vessels is difficult. In cirrhotic livers, more careful transection and hemostasis are required. With a careful CC technique, LigaSure™ can be used safely in patients with cirrhotic liver [9].

References

1. Gurusamy KS, Pamecha V, Sharma D, Davidson BR (2009) Techniques for liver parenchymal transection in liver resection. Cochrane database of systematic rev (Online) (1):CD006880
2. Palazzo FF, Francis DL, Clifton MA (2002) Randomized clinical trial of Ligasure versus open haemorrhoidectomy. Br J Surg 89(2):154–157
3. Jayne DG, Botterill I, Ambrose NS, Brennan TG, Guillou PJ, O'Riordain DS (2002) Randomized clinical trial of Ligasure versus conventional diathermy for day-case haemorrhoidectomy. Br J Surg 89(4):428–432
4. Lee WJ, Chen TC, Lai IR, Wang W, Huang MT (2003) Randomized clinical trial of Ligasure versus conventional surgery for extended gastric cancer resection. Br J Surg 90(12):1493–1496
5. Saiura A, Yamamoto J, Koga R, Sakamoto Y, Kokudo N, Seki M, Yamaguchi T, Yamaguchi T, Muto T, Makuuchi M (2006) Usefulness of LigaSure for liver resection: analysis by randomized clinical trial. Am J Surg 192(1):41–45
6. Ikeda M, Hasegawa K, Sano K, Imamura H, Beck Y, Sugawara Y, Kokudo N, Makuuchi M (2009) The vessel sealing system (LigaSure) in hepatic resection: a randomized controlled trial. Ann Surg 250(2):199–203
7. Patrlj L, Tuorto S, Fong Y (2010) Combined blunt-clamp dissection and LigaSure ligation for hepatic parenchyma dissection: postcoagulation technique. J Am Coll Surg 210(1):39–44
8. Romano F, Franciosi C, Caprotti R, Uggeri F, Uggeri F (2005) Hepatic surgery using the Ligasure vessel sealing system. World J Surg 29(1):110–112
9. Saiura A, Yamamoto J, Koga R, Seki M, Yamaguchi T (2008) Liver transection using the LigaSure sealing system. HPB (Oxford) 10(4):239–243

References

1. Sugarbaker DJ, Mentzer SJ (1992) Improved technique for hilar vascular stapling. Ann Thorac Surg 53:165–166
2. Nanashima A, Sumida Y, Oikawa M, Murakami G, Abo T, Hidaka S, Takeshita H, Sawai T, Nagayasu T (2009) Vascular transection using endovascular stapling in hepatic resection. Hepatogastroenterology 56:498–500
3. Fong Y, Blumgart LH (1997) Useful stapling techniques in liver surgery. J Am Coll Surg 185:93–100
4. Lefor AT, Flowers JL (1994) Laparoscopic wedge biopsy of the liver. J Am Coll Surg 178:307–308
5. Trede M (1993) Use of a laparoscopic disposable surgical stapler in liver resection. Chirurg 64:406–407
6. Zilling T, Walther BS, Holmin T (1990) Segmental liver resection with linear stapling device. An experimental study on pigs. In Vivo 4:273–275
7. Schemmer P, Bruns H, Weitz J, Schmidt J, Büchler M (2008) Liver transection using vascular stapler: a review. HPB (Oxford) 10:249–252
8. Schemmer P, Friess H, Dervenis C, Schmidt J, Weitz J, Uhl W, Büchler M (2007) The use of endo-GIA vascular staplers in liver surgery and their potential benefit: a review. Dig Surg 24:300–305
9. Schemmer P, Friess H, Hinz U, Mehrabi A, Kraus T, Z'graggen K, Schmidt J, Uhl W, Büchler M (2006) Stapler hepatectomy is a safe dissection technique: analysis of 300 patients. World J Surg 30:419–430
10. Poon R (2007) Current techniques of liver transection. HPB (Oxford) 9:166–173
11. Reddy S, Barbas A, Gan T, Hill S, Roche A, Clary B (2008) Hepatic parenchymal transection with vascular staplers: a comparative analysis with the crush-clamp technique. Am J Surg 196:760–767
12. Wang W, Fan S (2003) Use of the Endo-GIA vascular stapler for hepatic resection. Asian J Surg 26:193–196
13. Shah A, Callaway M, Thomas M, Finch-Jones M (2010) Contrast-enhanced intraoperative ultrasound improves detection of liver metastases during surgery for primary colorectal cancer. HPB (Oxford) 12:181–187
14. Li J, Malago M, Sotiropoulos G, Lang H, Schaffer R, Paul A, Broelsch C, Nadalin S (2009) Intraoperative application of "white test" to reduce postoperative bile leak after major liver resection: results of a prospective cohort study in 137 patients. Langenbecks Arch Surg 394:1019–1024
15. Nadalin S, Li J, Lang H, Sotiropoulos G, Schaffer R, Radtke A, Saner F, Broelsch C, Malago M (2008) The White test: a new dye test for intraoperative detection of bile leakage during major liver resection. Arch Surg 143:402–404 (discussion 404)
16. Chen X, Qiu F (2008) A simple technique ligating the corresponding inflow and outflow vessels during anatomical left hepatectomy. Langenbecks Arch Surg 393:227–230 (discussion 231–234)
17. Elias D, Dube P, Bonvalot S, Debanne B, Plaud B, Lasser P (1998) Intermittent complete vascular exclusion of the liver during hepatectomy: technique and indications. Hepatogastroenterology 45:389–395
18. Wu C, Yeh D, Ho W, Yu C, Cheng S, Liu T, P'eng F (2002) Occlusion of hepatic blood inflow for complex central liver resections in cirrhotic patients: a randomized comparison of hemihepatic and total hepatic occlusion techniques. Arch Surg 137:1369–1376
19. Rahbari NN, Zimmermann JB, Koch M, Bruckner T, Schmidt T, Elbers H, Reissfelder C, Weigand MA, Büchler MW, Weitz J (2009) IVC CLAMP: infrahepatic inferior vena cava clamping during hepatectomy—a randomised controlled trial in an interdisciplinary setting. Trials 10:94
20. Rahbari NN, Wente MN, Schemmer P, Diener MK, Hoffmann K, Motschall E, Schmidt J, Weitz J, Büchler MW (2008) Systematic review and meta-analysis of the effect of portal triad clamping on outcome after hepatic resection. Br J Surg 95:424–432

21. Balaa FK, Gamblin TC, Tsung A, Marsh JW, Geller DA (2008) Right hepatic lobectomy using the staple technique in 101 patients. J Gastrointest Surg 12:338–343
22. Jarnagin WR, Gonen M, Fong Y, DeMatteo RP, Ben-Porat L, Little S, Corvera C, Weber S, Blumgart LH (1803) Improvement in perioperative outcome after hepatic resection. Analysis of,consecutive cases over the past decade. Ann Surg 2002(236):397–407
23. Scheele J, Stangl R, Altendorf-Hofmann A, Paul M (1995) Resection of colorectal liver metastases. World J Surg 19:59–71
24. Fan ST, Lo CM, Liu CL, Lam CM, Yuen WK, Yeung C, Wong J (1999) Hepatectomy for hepatocellular carcinoma: toward zero hospital deaths. Ann Surg 229:322–330
25. Bruns H, Krätschmer K, Hinz U, Brechtel A, Keller M, Büchler M, Schemmer P (2010) Quality of life after curative liver resection: a single center analysis. World J Gastroenterol 16:2388–2395
26. Nicoud IB, Jones CM, Pierce JM, Earl TM, Matrisian LM, Chari RS, Gorden DL (2007) Warm hepatic ischemia-reperfusion promotes growth of colorectal carcinoma micrometastases in mouse liver via matrix metalloproteinase-9 induction. Cancer Res 67:2720–2728
27. van der Bilt JDW, Kranenburg O, Verheem A, van Hillegersberg R, BorelRinkes IHM (2006) Selective portal clamping to minimize hepatic ischaemia-reperfusion damage and avoid accelerated outgrowth of experimental colorectal liver metastases. Br J Surg 93:1015–1022
28. Nijkamp MW, van der Bilt JD, Snoeren N, Hoogwater FJ, van Houdt WJ, Molenaar IQ, Kranenburg O, van Hillegersberg R, Borel Rinkes IH (2010) Prolonged portal triad clamping during liver surgery for colorectal liver metastases is associated with decreased time to hepatic tumour recurrence. Eur J Surg Oncol 36(2):182–188
29. Hoffmann K, Franz C, Hinz U, Schirmacher P, Herfarth C, Eichbaum M, Büchler MW, Schemmer P (2010) Liver resection for multimodal treatment of breast cancer metastases: identification of prognostic factors. Ann Surg Oncol 17(6):1546–1554

Fusion Technique for Liver Transection: A New Technique Combining Kelly-Clysis and Harmonic Technology

11

Palepu Jagannath, Deepak Chhabra and Rajiv Shah

11.1 Introduction

The two important steps in liver transection involve: (1) splitting the liver parenchyma and (2) securing hemostasis. Traditional finger fracture (digitoclasy) for splitting the liver parenchyma is no longer practiced, and the widely used liver splitting techniques include clamp–crushing (Kelly-clysis), Cavitron ultrasonic surgical aspirator (CUSA; Integra Radionics), ultrasonic dissector (UD), or Hydro-jet®. Once the liver is split, securing hemostasis is critical and the exposed blood vessels and/or smaller biliary radicals are divided after suture ligation, bipolar coagulation or hemoclip application. With progress in energy devices, many new instruments are now available with the capability to seal hepatic vessels during parenchymal transection [1, 2]. These instruments are used in two approaches: (a) precoagulation technique and (b) postcoagulation technique.

Electronic Supplementary Material The online version of this article (doi:10.1007/978-88-470-2622-3_11) contains supplementary material which is available to authorized users.

P. Jagannath (✉) · D. Chhabra · R. Shah
Department of Surgical Oncology, Lilavati Hospital and Research Centre, Mumbai, Maharashtra, India
e-mail: drjagannath@gmail.com

D. Chhabra
e-mail: drdeepakchhbra@gmail.com

R. Shah
e-mail: drshahrajiv@gmail.com

I. Di Carlo (ed.), *Open, Laparoscopic and Robotic Hepatic Transection*,
DOI: 10.1007/978-88-470-2622-3_11, © Springer-Verlag Italia 2012

In the precoagulation technique, the energy devices use the principles of radiofrequency ablation or bipolar coagulation that burn and seal the hepatic parenchyma before transection. In the postcoagulation technique, the liver is split and then harmonic technology or bipolar coagulation is used for sealing the vessels utilizing another device. The devices used in a precoagulation strategy include RF-HABIB 4x, TissueLink®, LigaSure®, and Gyrus® forceps. All these devices need another instrument for cutting the precoagulated liver parenchyma [1]. The large vessels remain poorly visualized in the precoagulated tissues and can bleed on transection. In addition, blood vessels or biliary radicals from adjacent parts of the liver meant to be salvaged can be inadvertently injured by this "blind" coagulation technique. Biliary leaks are frequent. Thus, none of the techniques are ideal.

An ideal technique should:

(a) Provide precise parenchymal dissection and simultaneous vessel coagulation
(b) Be cost effective with a short learning curve.

The instrument for such a technique should:

(a) Be easy to assemble and use
(b) Be comfortable to handle (i.e., ergonomically convenient)
(c) Facilitate dissection around the larger vascular pedicles
(d) Have the ability to follow a curved transection path if needed
(e) Be a single instrument instead of multiple expensive devices crowding the operating room.

We have introduced a fusion technique (FT) or "Focus-clysis" which is a combination of Kelly-clysis and Harmonic technology as a precise technique for liver transection, combining both steps, i.e., parenchymal split and hemostasis, with one instrument, with the advantage of negligible lateral parenchymal damage.

11.2 Device Description

The instrument used for the FT is the Harmonic Focus® curved shears, which weighs just over 110 g. This device is a Kelly clamp-like instrument and consists of a soft-grip, scissor-handle housing assembly with two hand controls for power levels (MIN for minimum power level and MAX for maximum power level). The instrument is available in two lengths: regular and long, with differing shaft lengths of 9 and 17 cm (for deeper access), respectively (Fig. 11.1). The curved shears have 16-mm-long blades with a unique jaw design for transecting, sealing, grasping, and dissection. One of the clamp arms is inactive to help protect tissue in contact with the shaft. The instrument is attached to a Harmonic generator and uses the Harmonic technology to control bleeding by coaptive coagulation at low temperatures ranging from 50 to 100 °C. The electrical energy produced by the generator passes into the handpiece, wherein piezoelectric ceramic discs convert electrical energy into mechanical motion. Mechanical motion is transferred to the shaft, where it is amplified by silicon nodes. The blade vibrates longitudinally at

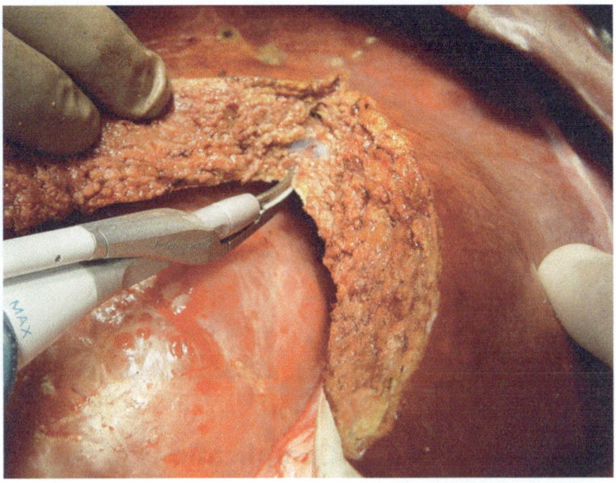

Fig. 11.1 Harmonic Focus® curved shears: long and short instruments

55,500 Hz, enabling tissue separation with minimal thermal transfer. Low-frequency ultrasonic energy creates cellular friction, causing amino acids in protein to unwind and reshape and hydrogen bonds to break. The amino acids transform into a new protein shape, forming a sticky coagulum that seals vessels.

11.3 Technique Description

The liver is mobilized as usual. Selective inflow occlusion is used according to surgeon preference. Once the line of demarcation is apparent, the Focus® instrument is used as a Kelly clamp at the edge of the liver (the starting point of the parenchymal split) with a gentle crush and simultaneous use of Harmonic technology to split approximately 1 cm of liver parenchyma. Subsequently, the capsule is cut by pushing the instrument immediately below it with gentle crush and simultaneous Harmonic technology to seal any underlying capsular vessels. The Focus® handpiece acts like a Kelly clamp that is held open with the tip approximately 0.5–1.0 cm apart, and splits the liver approximately 1 cm at a time. The curved tapered tips of the instrument allow precise dissection, and the parenchyma is split using the gentle clamp–crush technique (Fig. 11.2), exposing the vascular structures. No instrument change is needed for coagulation or cutting. The precision of cutting and coagulation is controlled by the surgeon by adjusting the power level and blade pressure. The controls on the handpiece are convenient for adjusting the coagulating power. Vessels of 1–2 mm are coagulated and transected at higher power, while those of 2–5 mm are coagulated and transected at low power. Vessels larger than 5 mm can be dissected and ligated. Minimal lateral thermal spread ($\leq$2 mm) allows for use near vital structures as well.

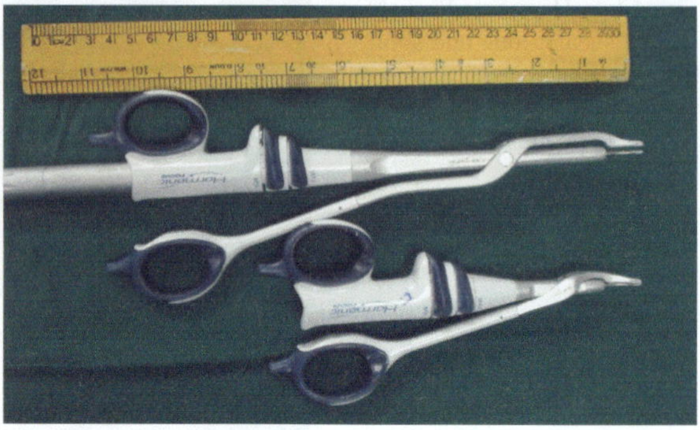

Fig. 11.2 Liver transection by FT (Focus-clysis)

11.3.1 Results and Complications

We have used the FT (Focus-clysis) for 52 consecutive hepatic resections (25 minor and 27 major resections). Indications for resections included hepatocellular carcinoma, intrahepatic and hilar cholangiocarcinoma, gallbladder carcinoma, neuroendocrine liver metastases, colorectal liver metastases, primary liver sarcomas, hepatoblastoma, and certain other metastatic tumors (Table 11.1). In our initial report [3], 18 consecutive noncirrhotic hepatic resections performed with FT were compared with 18 consecutive patients operated with UD (CUSA) prior to the availability of this technique (Table 11.2). The numbers of minor hepatic resections (<3 segments) and major hepatic resections (≥ 3 segments) were similar in both groups. Adequacy of remnant liver was assessed by preoperative computed tomography (CT) volumetric analysis. A Glissonian pedicle approach was used where feasible with selective inflow occlusion during transection. A postresection intraoperative cholangiogram was done in all major liver resections to check for bile leak. No additional methods of reinforcing hemostasis such as cellulose-gelatine preparations or spraying the cut surface with fibrin glue were used. Postoperative liver function was determined 24 h after the resection, and all clinically significant postoperative biliary leaks were documented with a hippuric iminodiacetic acid (HIDA) scan.

1. *FT resulted in a faster parenchymal split*

Though Kelly-clysis is one of the faster means of parenchymal transection, it requires an additional coagulating instrument. Although the time taken for liver split is not a criterion for the end result, Focus-clysis is similar to Kelly-clysis for parenchymal splitting. Additionally, the simultaneous coagulating property obviates the need for any instrument exchange for coagulation. Our first liver transection with the new instrument (Focus®) took 50 min; our subsequent major resections lasted for an average of only 25 min. The transection times with our earlier technique using CUSA and bipolar coagulation ranged from 35 to 80 min for major liver resections (Table 11.2).

Table 11.1 Demographics of patients with liver resections by FT

Fusion technique	
Patients, *n*	52
Gender, male/female	27/24
Age (years), median (range)	54 (3–74)
Indication for resection	
Hepatocellular carcinoma	11
Colorectal liver metastases	14
Neuroendocrine liver metastases	5
Cholangiocarcinoma	6
Gallbladder carcinoma	9
Primary liver sarcoma	2
Hepatoblastoma	1
Other metastatic	2
Benign	1
Resections	
Minor ($n = 25$)	
Left lateral segment resections	4
Right posterior sectionectomy	1
Segmentectomy	2
Multiple segmentectomy	2
Wedge resections (seg. 4b + 5 excision)	8
Metastasectomy	8
Major ($n = 27$)	
Central resections	3
Lobectomy	23
Extended resections	1
Complications	
Biliary fistula	3
Hepatic insufficiency	1
Others	6
Mortality	1

Table 11.2 Patient characteristics in the FT and ultrasonic dissection-bipolar coagulation (CUSA) liver resection group (6)

	Fusion technique	CUSA-bipolar group
Patients, *n*	18	18
Gender, male/female	7/11	9/9
Age (years), mean (range)	50.6 (19–74)	59.3 (42–71)
Pre-operative risk evaluation		
ASA score 1/2/3	12/6/0	6/11/1
Indication for resection		
Hepatocellular carcinoma	3	3
Colorectal liver metastases	6	5
Neuroendocrine tumors	1	2
Cholangiocarcinoma	3	4
Gallbladder carcinoma	3	4
Other liver tumors	2	Nil
Type of liver resection		
Major (≥3 segments)	9	9
Minor (<3 segments)	9	9
Surgery type, n		
Right hemihepatectomy	3	2
Left hemihepatectomy	3	2
Left hemihepatectomy + caudate lobectomy	1	2
Left extended hepatectomy	0	2
Right posterior sectionectomy	0	1
Left lateral sectionectomy	2	1
Segment 4b + 5 resection	3	5
Central (median) hepatectomy	2	1
Nonanatomical resections	4	2
Outcome data		
Mean blood loss overall ml (range)	416 (50–1,000)	833 (200–2,400)
Patients receiving RBC transfusion in first 48 h, *n*	2	8
Average transection time, min (range)	15–50	35–80

(continued)

Table 11.2 (continued)

	Fusion technique	CUSA-bipolar group
Morbidity		
Biliary fistula	1	4
Hepatic insufficiency	0	1
Others	3	6
Post-op Liver Functions		
Mean AST levels, (IU/L)	305.75	391.33
Mean ALT levels, (IU/L)	267.75	436.4
Mean Alk PO_4 level, (IU/L)	83.08	131.46

Abbreviations: *ASA* American Society of Anesthesiologists; *AST* aspartate aminotransferase; *ALT* alanine aminotransferase; *Alk* PO_4 alkaline phosphatase; *RBC* red blood cells

2. *Excellent hemostasis was achieved with FT without any instrument exchange*
   All intrahepatic portal venous branches, hepatic venous tributaries, and short direct tributaries from caudate lobe to IVC up to 5 mm could be securely coagulated using Focus®. Ligatures were limited only to right inferior hepatic vein (if encountered) or large tributaries of middle hepatic vein. No hemoclips were used. Also, there were no cases complicated by postoperative hemorrhage.
3. *FT was related with lower blood loss*
   The overall mean blood loss was lower in the FT group (416 ml; range 50–1,000 ml) compared with the CUSA group (833 ml; range 200–2,400 ml). Consequently, the postoperative transfusion requirements were lower in the FT group (11 versus 44 % in the CUSA-bipolar group). Only two patients required blood transfusion in the FT group compared with eight patients in the CUSA group.
4. *Biliary leaks were lower with the FT*
   Smaller biliary ducts could be selectively identified, ligated, and secured with the precision of clamp–crushing with the Focus®. Only one patient had a bile leak in the FT group compared with four patients in the CUSA group. Three other patients had complications in the FT group; however, they were unrelated to the technique used, including streptococcal bacteremia, surgical-site infection, and lung consolidation, respectively.
5. *No major derangements were noted in postoperative liver functions with the FT*
   Lower mean postoperative aspartate aminotransferase, alanine aminotransferase, and alkaline phosphatase levels indicated minimal lateral tissue damage during liver transection with FT; however, other biochemical liver parameters were comparable to in the CUSA group.

Our initial parenchymal transections were performed with the short regular Focus® hand probe, and it was technically more tedious to split the liver at depth, especially in large livers, in obese patients, and in patients with narrow costal margins that precluded adequate exposure. This technical difficulty was overcome in subsequent liver resections that were performed with the long hand probe.

Complications in our cohort of 52 patients included three biliary leaks (5.7 %), two of which were managed conservatively while one patient required stenting. One patient died due to hepatic insufficiency related to small liver remnant, not a complication of the technique per se. Complications in three other patients included streptococcal bacteremia, surgical-site infection, and lung consolidation. All remaining patients had better functional outcomes with FT.

11.4 Conclusions

Focus-clysis (FT) using a combination similar to Kelly-clysis and Harmonic technology is a promising, easy, and effective postcoagulation technique for liver transection, especially in noncirrhotic patients. The effect(s) of this device in cirrhotic livers has not been defined or addressed. Our initial results have shown advantages over the routinely used CUSA–bipolar combination, while our subsequent clinical experience demonstrates an acceptable safety and performance profile for its use in all types of hepatic resection.

References

1. McGahan JP, Khatri VP (2008) Imaging findings after liver resection by using radiofrequency parenchymal coagulation devices: initial experiences. Radiology 247:896–902
2. Campagnacci R, De SA, Baldarelli M et al. (2007) Hepatic resections by means of electrothermal bipolar vessel device (EBVS) LigaSure V: early experience. Surg Endosc 21:2280–2284
3. Jagannath P, Chhabra DG, Sutariya KR, Shah RC (2010) Fusion technique for liver transection with Kelly-clysis and harmonic technology. World J Surg 1(34):101–105

Ultrasound-Guided Delimitation of the Resection Area

12

Matteo Donadon and Guido Torzilli

12.1 Introduction

Performance of hepatic surgery without a parenchyma-sparing strategy carries significant risks for patient survival because of the nonnegligible occurrence of postoperative liver failure [1]. A key factor in modern hepatic surgery is use of intraoperative ultrasound (IOUS) not only to stage the disease but more importantly to guide resection. Whether in patients with hepatocellular carcinoma and underlying liver cirrhosis or in patients with colorectal liver metastasis, IOUS allows the performance of so-called conservative but radical surgery [2], which is the pivotal factor offering a chance of cure to an increasing proportion of patients, who until a few years ago were considered only for palliative care. Starting from some outlines of operative techniques in liver surgery, this chapter describes specifically the techniques for open hepatic transection using some crucial IOUS findings to define the area of resection.

12.2 Outlines of Operative Techniques for Liver Resection

The operative technique for liver resection is based on the segmental hepatic anatomy described by Couinaud in 1957, while the current nomenclature used for anatomic resection was updated in the Brisbane meeting in 2000. Generally, the operation starts with a J-shaped laparotomy, which can be extended with a thoracotomy in the ninth intercostal space for those patients with tumors close to

G. Torzilli (✉)
Liver Surgery Unit, Department of General Surgery, University of Milan,
IRCCS Istituto Clinico Humanitas, Milan, Italy
e-mail: guido.torzilli@humanitas.it, guido.torzilli@unimi.it

I. Di Carlo (ed.), *Open, Laparoscopic and Robotic Hepatic Transection*,
DOI: 10.1007/978-88-470-2622-3_12, © Springer-Verlag Italia 2012

the hepatocaval confluence. After full exploration of the peritoneal cavity, the liver is partially mobilized by dividing the round and falciform ligament. Pulling the round ligament, the liver is inspected, palpated, and more importantly evaluated by IOUS. Usually, the resection is carried out with low central venous pressure, using control of inflow (Pringle's maneuver) and sometimes of outflow by clamping of hepatic vein (HV) at the caval confluence.

12.2.1 IOUS of the Liver

IOUS is the procedure of choice to stage the disease in patients with liver tumors. It should be fully performed by the surgeon in charge of the operation rather than by assistants, radiologists, or technicians. This is because information gathered during the exploration requires interpretation to be most profitable with the aim of impacting on the surgical strategy. Generally, high-frequency probes (7.5–10 MHz) are recommended to perform IOUS, since they allow for higher spatial resolution than those working at lower frequencies (3.5–5 MHz). However, those latter probes are very useful for initial exploration, providing a better panoramic view. Lower-frequency probes are also useful for allowing contrast-enhanced intraoperative ultrasonography. Different shapes of probes are available for intraoperative use: linear T-shaped, interdigital, and microconvex probes. The best probe is the one that ensures the optimal compromise between the volume of the probe itself, which should be minimal, the scanning windows, which should be the largest, and stability once in contact with the liver surface. In this sense, a new microlinear probe with trapezoid scanning windows represents probably the best compromise among all the aforementioned requirements; this probe is furthermore designed to meet the requirements for the maneuvers as discussed in this chapter (Fig. 12.1).

12.2.2 Resection Guidance

Apart from staging, IOUS is essential to guide resection. It is almost impossible to correctly define the hepatic segmental boundaries without IOUS, as well as the boundaries of the tumor itself, because of the existing wide variations in anatomy. The main advantage of IOUS-guided resection is the modification of the traditional approach to liver tissue dissection, which involves dissection in vertical planes to avoid tumor exposure on the cut surface. With IOUS, the relationship between the dissection plane and the tumor edge can be followed in real time, and the direction of the dissection plane can be modified when needed. Versatile dissection planes around the tumors can avoid tumor exposure while sparing important vascular structures. This approach has been recently redefined by the authors as the "radical but conservative approach" and should be applied in liver surgery to provide the best results [2]. Also in patients in whom major resections are required, IOUS allows better design of the dissection plane, leading to conservative surgery even

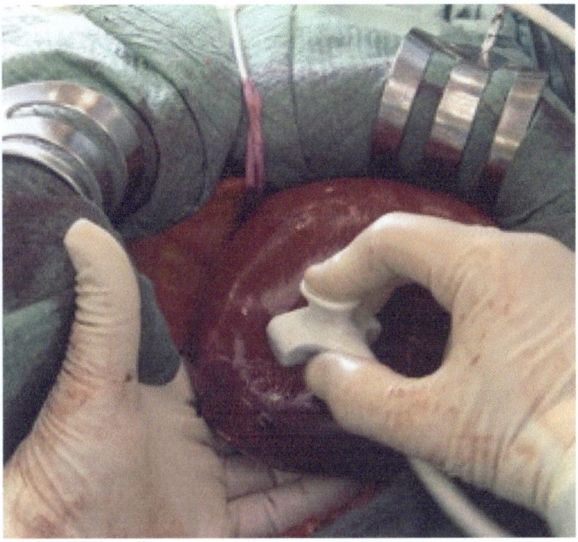

Fig. 12.1 Most recent personally designed probe for IOUS. Of note, this probe has a trapezoid scanning area, and an ergonomic shape, which may help during IOUS-guided maneuvers

in case of complex presentation [3]. Specific and original IOUS techniques have already been developed to help the surgeon during the operation [4–6]. The following paragraphs focus on two crucial techniques for defining the area of resection using IOUS findings.

12.3 Anatomical Resection by Ultrasound-Guided Finger Compression

Initially used for tumors located in the left hemiliver [6], more recently application of this method has been successfully extended to any segment [7], including segment 8, and even to sectional portion of the liver [8]. Once the feeding portal branch is identified by IOUS, it can be compressed using the IOUS probe on one side of the liver and the finger on the opposite side (Fig. 12.2) with the aim of inducing transient ischemia of the portion of the liver distal to the compression site. This portion can then be marked by electrocautery, the compression be released, and the resection be carried out. This technique is simple, fast, noninvasive, and reversible. Moreover, the possibility to modify the site of compression and then the resection volume allows tailoring of the resection as a function of tumor features and the status of the background liver. However, the compression can be used in a counter-compression perspective that is the definition of the adjacent segmental margins to disclose the margins of the segment to be removed. Indeed for segments such as segments 1 and 4 superior for which direct compression of the feeding portal branch could result infeasible for anatomical reasons, the compression of the adjacent segmental branches allows definition of their segmental margins.

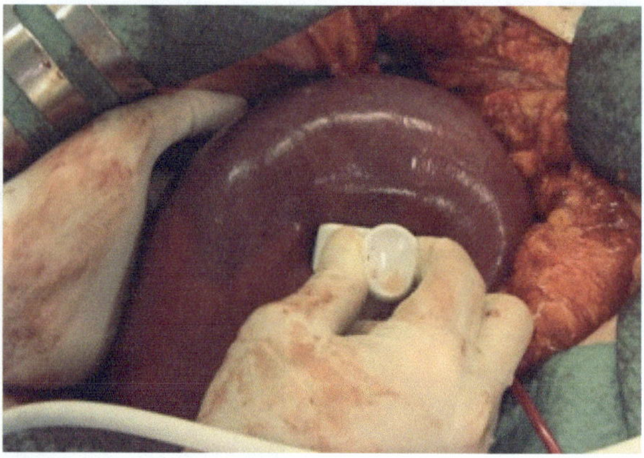

Fig. 12.2 Ischemic demarcation by ultrasound-guided finger compression technique in a patient with HCC in segment 8. The probe is handled with the right hand, while with the left hand the surgeon compresses the target pedicle

12.4 Tailoring the Area of Resection Using Outflow Findings

The area of resection may be tailored not only using ultrasound-guided finger compression of portal branch as described above, but also using the IOUS findings of the outflow control. Indeed, we have already shown how to minimize sacrifice of liver parenchyma even in those patients with tumor at the hepatocaval confluence, for which standard major or extended hepatectomy should be indicated. Moreover, we have introduced some new operations, such as the *mini-mesohepatectomy* and the *systematic extended right sectionectomy* [9, 10], which simultaneously limit the need for formal major resection and improve the chances of resection for those patients with complex tumoral presentation. The definition of the resection area using the outflow control is based on extensive use of IOUS flow analyses, with the aim of checking the outflow modifications once a HV which should be resected for oncological reasons is clamped; for this purpose, other than its encirclement, the surgeon's fingertip compression at caval confluence guided by ultrasound could be enough. At that time, the search is focused at least on one of the following: reversal flow direction in the peripheral portion of the compressed HV, which suggests drainage through collateral circulation in adjacent HVs or inferior vena cava (IVC); detectable shunting collaterals between the compressed HV and adjacent HV or IVC (Fig. 12.3); hepatopetal flow in the portal branch(es) corresponding to the area drained by the compressed HV. Using these criteria, the area of resection may be really tailored and individualized based on the tumoral presentation and liver background of each patient, minimizing the rate of major or extended resection and thus related morbidity and mortality rates.

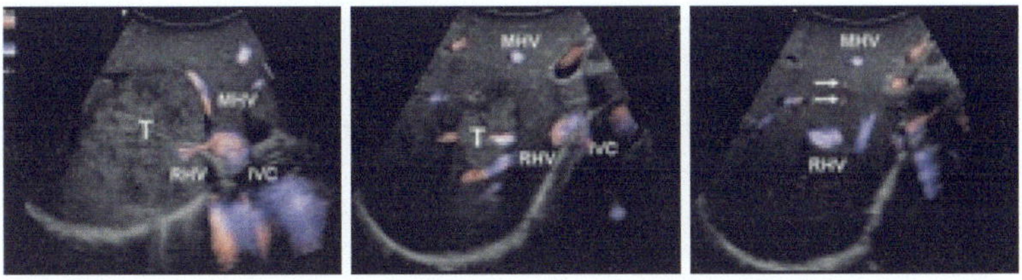

Fig. 12.3 Collateral veins (*arrows*) between the right hepatic vein (*RHV*) and the middle hepatic vein (*MHV*) in a patient with large colorectal metastasis involving the RHV at its caval confluence

12.5 Conclusions

IOUS is the best method for staging liver involvement by the tumor, and it is certainly the best method for the surgeon to understand in real time the liver anatomy and the relations between tumors and intrahepatic vessels, thus enabling performance of effective surgical operations. IOUS guidance allows expansion of indications, offering the chance of cure to a greater proportion of patients who would otherwise be excluded from the surgical program or submitted to more traditional but riskier operations.

References

1. Vauthey JN, Pawlik TM, Abdalla EK et al (2004) Is extended hepatectomy for hepatobiliary malignancy justified? Ann Surg 239:722–739
2. Torzilli G, Montorsi M, Donadon M et al (2005) "Radical but conservative" is the main goal for ultrasonography-guided liver resection: prospective validation of this approach. J Am Coll Surg 201:517–528
3. Torzilli G, Procopio F, Botea F et al (2009) One-stage ultrasonographically guided hepatectomy for multiple bilobar colorectal metastases: a feasible and effective alternative to the 2-stage approach. Surgery 146:60–71
4. Makuuchi M, Hasegawa H, Yamazaki S (1985) Ultrasonically guided subsegmentectomy. Surg Gynecol Obstet 161:346–350
5. Torzilli G, Montorsi M, Del Fabbro D et al (2006) Ultrasonographically guided surgical approach to liver tumors involving the hepatic veins close to the caval confluence. Br J Surg 93:1238–1246
6. Torzilli G, Makuuchi M (2004) Ultrasound-guided finger compression in liver subsegmentectomy for hepatocellular carcinoma. Surg Endosc 18:136–139
7. Torzilli G, Procopio F, Cimino M et al (2010) Anatomical segmental and subsegmental resection of the liver for hepatocellular carcinoma: a new approach by means of ultrasound-guided vessel compression. Ann Surg 251:229–235
8. Torzilli G, Procopio F, Palmisano A et al (2009) New technique for defining the right anterior section intraoperatively using ultrasound-guided finger counter-compression. J Am Coll Surg 209:e8–11

9. Torzilli G, Donadon M, Marconi M et al (2008) Systematic extended right posterior sectionectomy: a safe and effective alternative to right hepatectomy. Ann Surg 247:603–611
10. Torzilli G, Palmisano A, Procopio F et al (2010) A new systematic small for size resection for liver tumors invading the middle hepatic vein at its caval confluence: the mini-mesohepatectomy. Ann Surg 251:33–39

Open Hepatic Transection Using Ultrasonic Dissector

13

Giorgio Ercolani, Matteo Ravaioli, Matteo Serenari, Paolo Di Gioia and Antonio Daniele Pinna

13.1 Introduction

Blood loss, subsequent blood transfusion, and operative time are strongly associated with perioperative morbidity, mortality, and poor long-term outcome [1]. The type of parenchymal transection might significant affect intraoperative bleeding. Hepatic parenchyma has been transected using several techniques that have evolved for liver surgery over the past years: Lin first described in 1958 the finger fracture technique [2], improved some years later by using Kelly or Péan clamps (clamp crushing) [3]. Newer instruments include ultrasound-based devices such as ultrasonic dissectors (UD) or ultrasonic shears (Harmonic Scalpel), water-jet dissectors, and radiofrequency dissecting sealers (TissueLink), whereas the role of stapling devices remains controversial and needs further investigation [4].

The clamp-crush technique is still the reference standard due to faster transection speed, lower blood loss, and being two to six times cheaper than other resection methods; a recent review dealing with types of technique and intraoperative

Electronic Supplementary Material The online version of this article (doi:10.1007/978-88-470-2622-3_13) contains supplementary material which is available to authorized users.

G. Ercolani (✉) · M. Ravaioli · M. Serenari · P. D. Gioia · A. D. Pinna
Department of Surgery and Transplantation, Sant'Orsola Hospital,
University of Bologna, Via Massarenti 9, 40138 Bologna, Italy
e-mail: giorgio.ercolani@aosp.bo.it

M. Ravaioli
e-mail: m.rava@hotmail.com

A. D. Pinna
e-mail: antoniodaniele.pinna@aosp.bo.it

I. Di Carlo (ed.), *Open, Laparoscopic and Robotic Hepatic Transection*,
DOI: 10.1007/978-88-470-2622-3_13,

bleeding did not reveal any advantages of new transection devices compared with the standard clamp-crush technique [5].

Nevertheless, ultrasonic dissector (CUSA, Sonosurg) has gained wide acceptance; it was first introduced as an instrument for parenchymal transection during hepatectomy by Hodgson and Del Guercio [6]; UD is a vibrating suction device that is able to remove liver parenchyma preferentially, dividing cells by the cavitational effect while causing minor injury to structures with high content of elastic tissues so that blood vessels and bile ducts can be dissected out cleanly, allowing safe ligation [7]. Thus, UD permits a blood-less operating field and excellent operating conditions to evaluate liver anatomy.

Randomized controlled trials have been published to compare clamp-crush and ultrasonic dissector, but there were no significant differences in mortality or morbidity rates [5, 8–10]. In particular, only one randomized study comparing CUSA without vascular occlusion and clamp-crush with vascular occlusion showed a significant increase of bleeding and amount of transfused patients in the group of CUSA [10]. On the contrary, in the trials where vascular control was applied equally between groups, no differences were found in terms of blood loss, number of transfused patients, or transection time between CUSA and other techniques [5, 8, 9].

13.2 Device Description

Sonosurg as well as CUSA (Sonosurg, SS, Olympus Medical Systems Corporation, Tokyo, Japan; or Cavitron Ultrasonic Surgical Aspirator, Tyco Healthcare, Mansfield, MA) are composed of a main generator, a transducer, and an irrigation/suction unit and probes for different uses with related sheaths (Fig. 13.1).

Ultrasonic waves, responsible for cutting parenchyma, are produced by passing electric energy through either piezoelectric or magnetic transducer. Its function is based on the physical principle of fragmentation of biological tissues by a probe vibrating at high frequencies (from 23 to 34 kHz). Irrigation by cooling water is required to prevent the probe from heating and causing damage, while the aspiration system must remove tissue debris and improve the quality of the surgical field, which should be cleared in order to clearly identify parenchymal structures.

The transducer to which the probe is attached has to be inserted into the sheath from the proximal end and pushed all the way in until it stops (Fig. 13.2). The irrigation/suction tube is connected properly to the transducer (Fig. 13.3) and to the pump head in order to ensure saline solution flow. Before attempting to emulsify tissue, it has to be confirmed that cooling water flows from the sheath tip. After liver capsule has been opened by diathermy, the sheath is applied at the proposed transection line. Suction pressure and rate of saline irrigation have to be properly set. It is indicated to start always with relatively low suction pressure and increase it gradually as required during use. The effect of tissue fragmentation is more intense in collagen-poor tissues and should be carried out selectively,

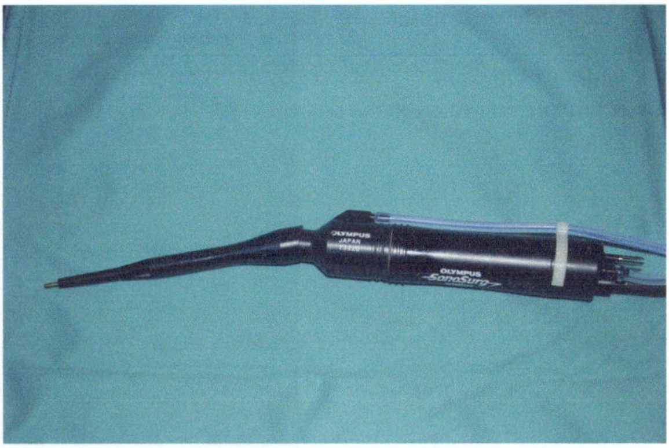

Fig. 13.1 The probe of ultrasonic dissector (the probe of Sonosurg and CUSA are quite similar)

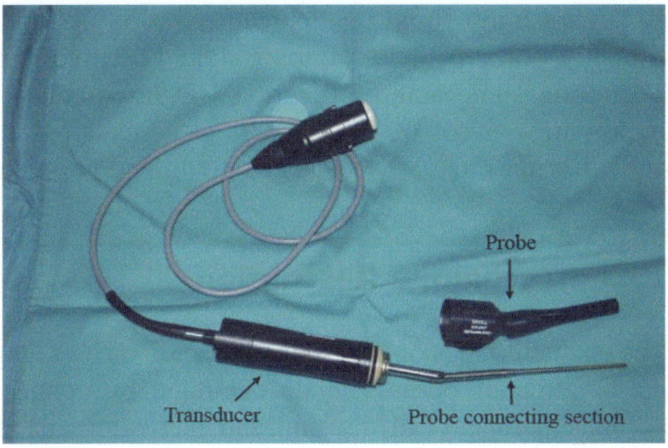

Fig. 13.2 The probe connection to transducer

avoiding biliary and vascular structures. Adjustment of the amplitude of the oscillations provides different power levels of tissue dissection. Lower levels are appropriate for normal hepatic parenchyma and higher levels for fibrotic liver. Indeed, if high suction pressure is used from the beginning, tissues may be easily damaged by aspiration or subjected to unexpected dissection, fragmentation, emulsification, or aspiration during ultrasonic treatment. As reported above, the device allows one to leave arteries, veins, and bile ducts, which can be cauterized by an assistant, whereas larger ones can be ligated or clipped. Moreover, blood loss, tissue debris, and injected saline can be cleared away by using an additional aspirator, which should always be available in the surgical field.

Thanks to its properties, ultrasonic dissector is preferred by many liver surgeons: UD is more precise for dissection of hepatic vein branches or when the tumor is located close to a major hepatic vein (Fig. 13.4); in this situation, UD is very useful in identifying the involved vein, preparing the vessel above and below the tumor, and providing the surgeon with the possibility to resect or preserve it according to intraoperative findings and the relation between the tumor and the vein.

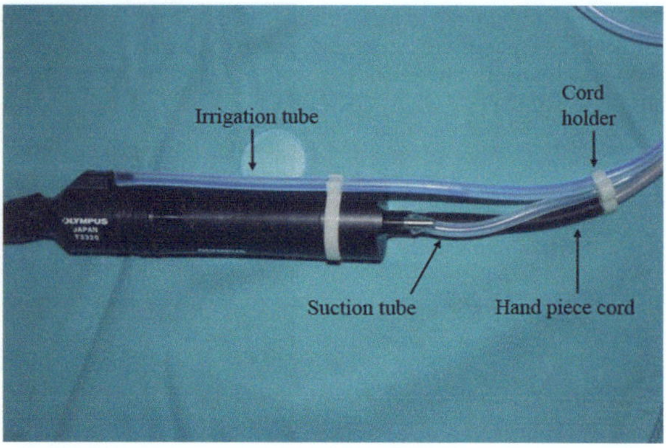

Fig. 13.3 The irrigation/suction tube is assembled on the probe of ultrasonic dissector and connected to the transducer

During transection, ligation/cauterization of small vessels and cautious application of portal pedicle clamping should be used to prevent massive bleeding [8]. Therefore, some authors describe UD in association with bipolar cautery, thus improving control of oozing and bleeding from the cut surface [7]. The low complication rate easily balances the high equipment costs in the long term.

13.3 Technique Description

The characteristics of ultrasonic dissector such as fragmentation of liver tissue and preservation of portal pedicle encircled by connective tissue are the basis for accurate parenchymal division and meticulous exposure of vascular and biliary pedicles, even if being unquestionably slower compared with other techniques.

The initial setting of the machine might be at 60–70 % power for ultrasonic dissection, and 50 % for suction (and irrigation). As already discussed, intermittent portal pedicle clamping is advisable to reduce intraoperative bleeding (15 min of clamping and 5 min of declamping is the standard method). During clamping, the UD is moved along the transection line (guided by intraoperative ultrasonography) with an "up-and-down" movement. Electrocoagulation is usually sufficient for small vessels, and metallic clip may also be used to close small hepatic veins. On the other hand, identification and meticulous ligature of larger vessels or small portal pedicles during transection is the best way to ensure hemostasis of the resected portion and to prevent intra- and postoperative bleeding. The resection should proceed slowly, with suction to remove tissue debris generated by UD during transection and to allow precise visualization of intraparenchymal structures.

During declamping, it is not advisable to proceed with transection, but a gauze should be placed along the line to prevent massive bleeding. Suture including small portion of parenchyma generally in Vicryl, or depending on type of surrounding parenchyma, complete hemostasis. Hemostasis may be problematic in cirrhotic livers or when the resected surface is uneven or vascular pedicles retract

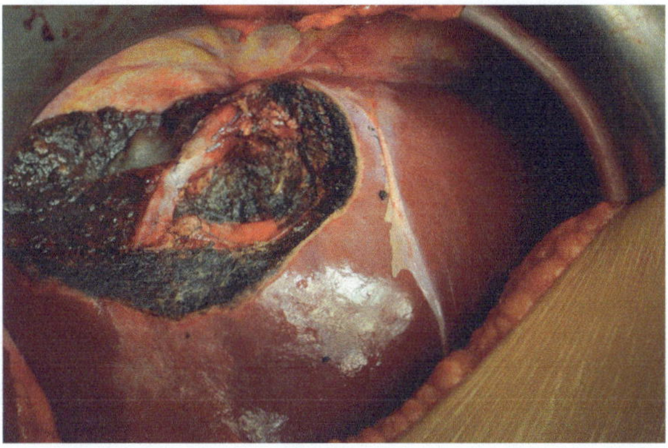

Fig. 13.4 Intraoperative finding after resection of large adenoma located between segment 7 and segment 8, adherent to right hepatic vein dissected by ultrasonic dissector

Table 13.1 Reported series of living-donor liver transplantation using CUSA for donor hepatectomy

Author	Year	City	No. of LDLT	Technique	PTC
Tanaka [12]	1993	Kyoto	760	UD + BC	No
Lo [13]	2000	Hong Kong	116	UD	NI
Malagò [14]	2003	Essen	74	UD + BC	NI
Broering [15]	2004	Hamburg	165	UD	NI
Shimul [16]	2006	Toronto	146	UD + HJD	NI
Hwang [17]	2006	Seoul	1000	UD + BC	No
Brown [18]	2008	New York	224	UD	Yes
Yaprak [19]	2011	Istanbul	181	UD	NI

NI no information, *PTC* portal triad clamping, *UD* ultrasonic dissector, *BC* bipolar cautery, *HJD* hydro-jet dissector

into the parenchyma. In these cases, wider suture stitches can be used (in these cases, 3/0 Prolene is often advisable).

Ultrasonic dissector is also the standard method in living-donor liver transplantation for donor hepatectomy. The shortage of cadaveric organs has led to an increase of this technique in the field of liver transplantation, with the first successful case reported by Strong in 1990 [11]. Thereafter, it was validated by other groups, and nowadays parenchymal transection is performed worldwide using ultrasonic dissector (Table 13.1). UD allows preservation of all vascular and biliary structures during transection of liver parenchyma; in particular, localization and control of not only the branches but also of the hepatic veins are more efficient. Since donor safety is the priority in LDLT, all efforts have to be made to spare the donor from operative hazards and postoperative complications. Even in this setting, most authors advocate additional use of bipolar cautery to coagulate peripheral fragile vessels and tiny hepatic veins to prevent late bleeding.

References

1. Gozzetti G, Mazziotti A, Grazi GL, Jovine E, Gallucci A, Gruttadauria S, Frena A, Morganti M, Ercolani G, Masetti M et al. (1995) Liver resection without blood transfusion. Br J Surg 82(8):1105–1110
2. Lin T, Tsu K, Mien C et al. (1958) Study on lobectomy of the liver. J Formosa Med Assoc 57:742–759
3. Lin TY (1974) A simplified technique for hepatic resection: the crush method. Ann Surg 180:285–290
4. Schemmer P, Friess H, Hinz U, Mehrabi A, Kraus TW, Z'graggen K, Schmidt J, Uhl W, Buchler MW (2006) Stapler hepatectomy is a safe dissection technique: analysis of 300 patients. World J Surg 30:419–430
5. Gurusamy KS, Pamecha V, Sharma D, Davidson BR (2009) Techniques for liver parenchymal transection in liver resection (review). Cochrane Libr 1:1–84
6. Hodgson WJB, DelGuercio LRM (1984) Preliminary experience in liver surgery using the ultrasonic scalpel. Surgery 95:203–204
7. Lesurtel M, Belghiti J (2008) Open hepatic parenchymal transection using ultrasonic dissection and bipolar coagulation. HPB (Oxford) 10(4):265–270
8. Takayama T, Makuuchi M, Kubota K, Harihara Y, Hui AM, Sano K et al. (2001) Randomized comparison of ultrasonic vs clamp transection of the liver. Arch Surg 136(8):922–928
9. Koo BN, Kil HK, Choi JS, Kim JY, Chun DH, Hong YW (2005) Hepatic resection by the Cavitron ultrasonic surgical aspirator increases the incidence and severity of venous air embolism. Anesth Analg 101(4):966–970, table of contents
10. Lesurtel M, Selzner M, Petrowsky H, McCormack L, Clavien PA (2005) How should transection of the liver be performed? A prospective randomized study in 100 consecutive patients: comparing four different transection strategies. Ann Surg 242(6):814–823
11. Strong RW, Lynch SV, Ong TH, Matsunami H, Koido Y, Balderson GA (1990) Successful liver transplantation from a living donor to her son. N Engl J Med 322:1505–1507
12. Tanaka K, Uemoto S, Tokunaga Y, Fujita S, Sano K, Nishizawa T, Sawada H, Shirahase I, Kim HJ, Yamaoka Y et al. (1993) Surgical techniques and innovations in living related liver transplantation. Ann Surg 217(1):82–91
13. Lo CM (2003) Complications and long-term outcome of living liver donors: a survey of 1,508 cases in five Asian centers. Transplantation 75:12
14. Malagó M, Testa G, Frilling A, Nadalin S, Valentin-Gamazo C, Paul A, Lang H, Treichel U, Cicinnati V, Gerken G, Broelsch CE (2003) Right living donor liver transplantation: an option for adult patients: single institution experience with 74 patients. Ann Surg 238(6):853–862, (discussion 862–863)
15. Broering DC, Wilms C, Bok P, Fischer L, Mueller L, Hillert C, Lenk C, Kim JS, Sterneck M, Schulz KH, Krupski G, Nierhaus A, Ameis D, Burdelski M, Rogiers X (2004) Evolution of donor morbidity in living related liver transplantation a single-center analysis of 165 cases. Ann Surg 240:1013–1026
16. Shimul A, Shah MD, Gary A, Levy MD, Lesley D, Adcock MD, Gary Gallagher RN, David R, Grant MD (2006) Adult-to-adult living donor liver transplantation. Can J Gastroenterol 20(5):339–343
17. Hwang S, Lee SG, Lee YJ, Sung KB, Park KM, Kim KH, Ahn CS, Moon DB, Hwang GS, Kim KM, Ha TY, Kim DS, Jung JP, Song GW (2006) Lessons learned from 1,000 living donor liver transplantations in a single center: how to make living donations safe. Liver Transpl 12(6):920–927
18. Brown RS Jr (2008) Live donors in liver transplantation. Gastroenterology 134(6):1802–1813

19. Yaprak O, Dayangac M, Demirbas T, Tabendeh B, Yuzer Y, Tokat Y (2011) Analysis of right lobe living-liver donor complications: a single center experience. Exp Clin Transplant 9(1):56–59

Part II
Laparoscopic Transection

14 Laparoscopic Hepatic Transection Using Microwave

Yuichiro Otsuka and Hironori Kaneko

14.1 Introduction

The Louisville Statement proposed recent opinion that laparoscopic hepatectomy (LH) is safe and effective in management of surgical liver disease, when performed by trained surgeons with experience in both hepatobiliary and laparoscopic surgery [1]. However, a major disadvantage of laparoscopic surgery as compared with open surgery is that it is not as well suited for addressing unexpected hemorrhaging during liver parenchymal transection. Therefore, the critical determinant for safe LH is thorough familiarity with laparoscopic instruments and equipment for maintenance of hemostasis [2].

Thermal ablation of the resection plane before liver parenchymal transection—using devices that are ideally suited for coagulation—is called precoagulation. We believe that use of a precoagulation technique performed by using devices that conduct radiofrequency or microwave energy helps reduce blood loss during parenchymal transection, especially in patients with liver cirrhosis [3].

Electronic Supplementary Material The online version of this article (doi:10.1007/978-88-470-2622-3_14) contains supplementary material which is available to authorized users.

Y. Otsuka · H. Kaneko (✉)
Department of Surgery (Omori), Toho University Faculty of Medicine, 6-11-1 Omori-nishi, Otaku, Tokyo 143-8541, Japan
e-mail: hironori@med.toho-u.ac.jp

Y. Otsuka
e-mail: yotsuka@med.toho-u.ac.jp

I. Di Carlo (ed.), *Open, Laparoscopic and Robotic Hepatic Transection*,
DOI: 10.1007/978-88-470-2622-3_14, © Springer-Verlag Italia 2012

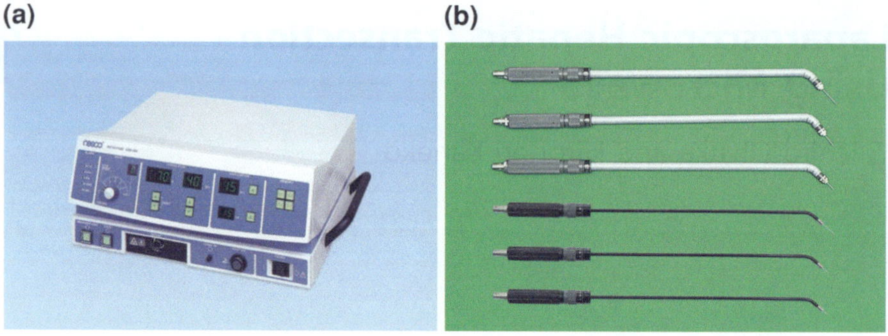

Fig. 14.1 The Microtaze AZM-550 generator (**a**), and microwave tissue coagulator probes (**b**) used in endoscopic surgery (Endo-Angle Probe®; Alfresa-Pharma Co., Inc., Osaka, Japan)

14.2 Device Description

The alternating radiative field used in microwave ablation causes polarized water molecules to oscillate. The agitation of water molecules generates friction, which causes heat and tissue destruction by coagulative necrosis. The Microtaze AZM-550 generator (Alfresa-Pharma Co, Inc., Osaka, Japan) emits microwaves at frequency of 2,450 MHz and wavelength of 12 cm and has a maximum output of 110 W. The emitted microwaves are transmitted to a reusable operating antenna via a coaxial cable (Fig. 14.1). As compared with radiofrequency devices, the absence of a ground patch on the patient's skin theoretically reduces the risk of burning. Currently available probes include a 5- to 10-mm diameter 45° flexible-angle probe with an 8-, 15-, or 20 mm needle antenna (Endo-Angle Probe®) in endoscopic surgery. For precoagulation in the superficial layer of the liver, the 5 mm Endo-Angle Probe® can be manipulated at the optimal point and angle through a single 5 mm trocar.

14.3 Technique Description

14.3.1 Basic Technique for Liver Parenchymal Transection Using Microwave Precoagulation

Laparoscopic liver resections are generally performed by using a 5- to 10-mm flexible-angle laparoscope with a four- or five-trocar technique. Laparoscopic flexible-angle ultrasonography is indispensable for assessing anatomic landmarks, such as the vasculobiliary connection and the surgical margins of the tumor. The line of intended liver parenchymal transection is marked on the liver surface using diathermy. The liver is punctured with the microwave needle probe along the line of transection and irradiated with microwaves (average power 75 watts for

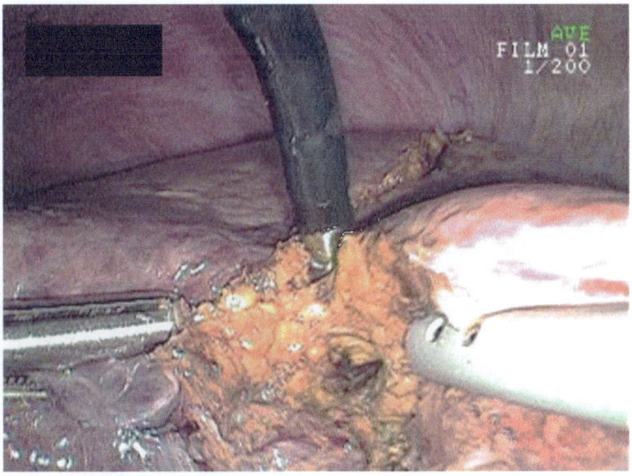

Fig. 14.2 Microwave precoagulation during pure laparoscopic right hemihepatectomy for hepatocellular carcinoma with chronic hepatitis

30 seconds at 1 cm intervals). Once resection of the liver surface is started using laparoscopic coagulating shears, exposed small vessels and biliary structures less than 2 mm in diameter are coagulated with a bipolar sealing system. Branched vessels greater than 2 mm in diameter are clipped and transected. Large vessels, including main Glisson's pedicles and major hepatic veins, can be divided using a laparoscopic linear stapler. However, care should be taken to avoid injury of the vessels when inserting the microwave needle electrode into the liver parenchyma. Therefore, saline-enhanced monopolar sealing devices are a better selection for precoagulation and hemostasis in deeper liver parenchyma.

Microwave also allows for a combination strategy (i.e., simultaneous tumor ablation with liver resection), even during laparoscopic procedures for multiple liver tumors. Pringle's maneuver is feasible laparoscopically but is usually unnecessary during these procedures.

14.3.2 Pure Laparoscopic Hepatectomy

Pure laparoscopic procedure is generally used in left lateral sectionectomy, and in partial hepatectomy for tumors located on the edge or surface of the inferolateral segments (segments II, III, IVb, V, and VI). The laparoscope is usually inserted at the periumbilicus. In partial hepatectomy, two or three trocars for manipulation are placed in a concentric circle radiating from the tumor. In left lateral sectionectomy, a trocar at epigastrium and additional two trocars at bilateral abdomen are placed. Liver parenchymal transection is performed using the technique mentioned above. With greater experience in laparoscopic liver resection, major hepatectomy, such as hemihepatectomy or other anatomical resection, can be performed with pure laparoscopic procedure, using five trocars (Figs. 14.2, 14.3). The specimen is usually retrieved from a suprapubic incision or a scar from a previous surgery.

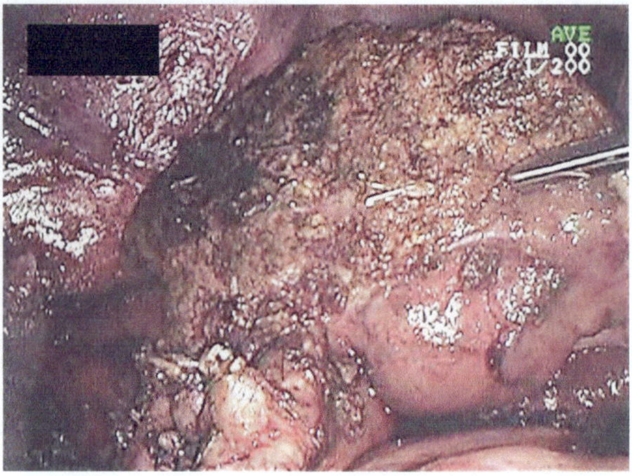

Fig. 14.3 Posttransection plane of pure laparoscopic right hemihepatectomy

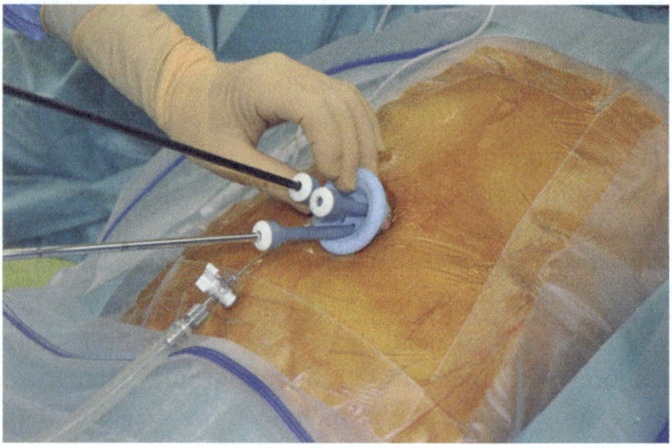

Fig. 14.4 SILS port system (Covidien, Inc., Boulder, CO, USA)

14.3.3 Single-Incision Laparoscopic Hepatectomy

In carefully selected patients, surgery is performed through a single supraumbilical port site, using a 25-mm SILS™ port (Covidien, Inc., Boulder, CO, USA) placed through an open approach. The incision is vertical and includes the umbilicus. A 5 mm deflectable-tip laparoscope (LTF-VH deflectable-tip video laparoscope; Olympus, Center Valley, PA, USA) is useful for this procedure. In general, three laparoscopic instruments are placed through the SILS port system (Fig. 14.4). Typically, a Roticulator™ Endo Grasp (Covidien, Inc.) is used straight or crossed to allow simultaneous traction. A microwave probe and the ultrasonic coagulating shears of a cutting instrument can be used via the other port. The microwave Endo-Angle Probe® permits precoagulation at the optimal point and angle, even in this limited working space (Fig. 14.5). The specimen is retrieved from the supraumbilical incision after resection is completed (Fig. 14.6).

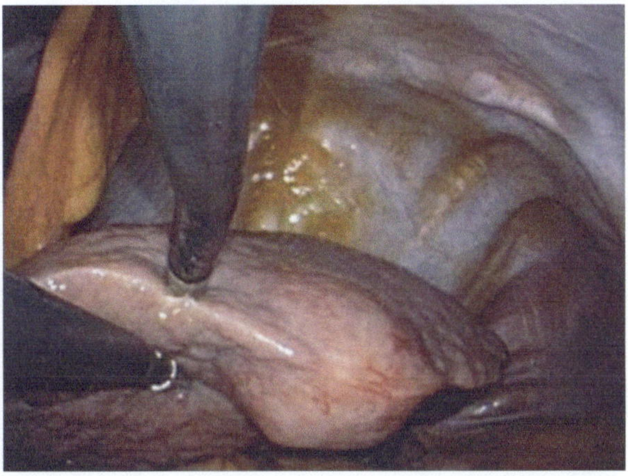

Fig. 14.5 Microwave precoagulation during single-incision laparoscopic partial hepatectomy in segment III for hepatocellular carcinoma with liver cirrhosis

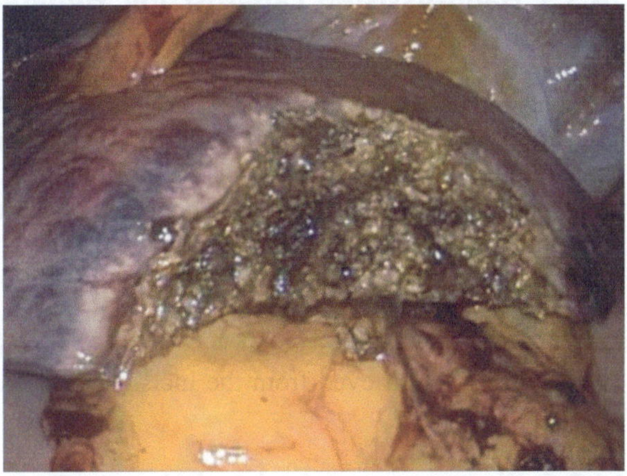

Fig. 14.6 Posttransection plane of single-incision laparoscopic partial hepatectomy

14.3.4 Laparoscopy-Assisted Hepatectomy

Laparoscopy-assisted hepatectomy, which is referred to as the hybrid procedure, has benefits for both open and laparoscopic procedures and can increase the indications and safety of minimally invasive liver resection [4]. In this procedure, liver parenchymal transection is performed through a small upper midline or subcostal laparotomy (7–12 cm skin incision) after laparoscopic mobilization of the liver with pneumoperitoneum. The same surgical maneuvers and instruments, as well as the microwave probe used in conventional open hepatectomy, are utilized through a minilaparotomy. Transection of the liver parenchyma under direct vision can be accomplished by elevating the transection line toward abdominal side by means of tape secured to the liver [5]. This technique is applicable to various types of resection, including anatomical hepatectomy and lymph node dissection of the hepatoduodenal ligament.

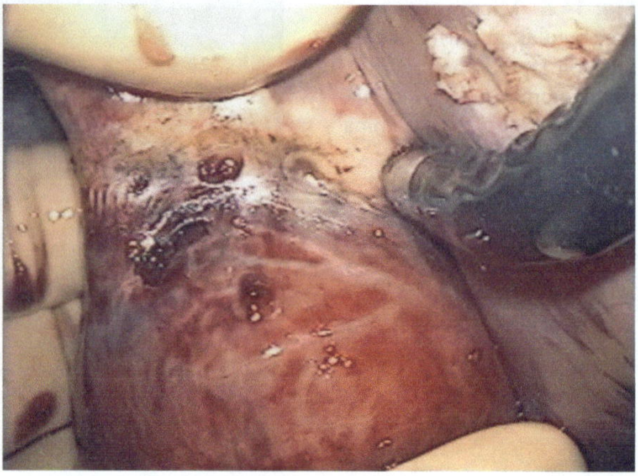

Fig. 14.7 Microwave precoagulation during hand-assisted partial liver resection of segment VII for hepatocellular carcinoma

14.3.5 Hand-Assisted Laparoscopic Hepatectomy

Hand-assisted LH is used for resection of tumors located in the posterosuperior segments of the liver (segments VII, VIII, and IVa). After mobilization of the right liver from the retroperitoneum and the surrounding ligament by laparoscopic procedure, an approximately 7-cm skin incision is made at the right lower quadrant to allow hand access for surgical maneuvers and extraction of the resected specimen through a LapDisk™ (Hakko Medical Industry, Tokyo, Japan). Use of the hand is also helpful for properly inserting the microwave Endo-Angle Probe® in the liver parenchyma, for verifying the tumor margin with retraction of the operative field, and for achieving hemostasis with compression (Figs. 14.7, 14.8). The specimen is retrieved from the incision used for hand access.

14.3.6 Thoracoscopy-Assisted Hepatectomy

Thoracoscopy-assisted technique is another option for resection of tumors located at the top of liver (e.g., segment VII or VIII) for which liver mobilization and retraction, as well as identification of tumor margins, are difficult to accomplish using a laparoscopic approach [6]. Microwave precoagulation technique using an Endo-Angle Probe® can be useful in overcoming the disadvantage of this approach, i.e., that Pringle's maneuver cannot be performed from the thoracic cavity to control intraoperative bleeding.

14.3.7 Complications and Results

Use of microwave technology in liver surgery was developed by Tabuse as a technique to minimize blood loss [7]. This technique has been followed by several groups in open hepatectomy [8, 9, 10]. In 1996, we described a novel technique in

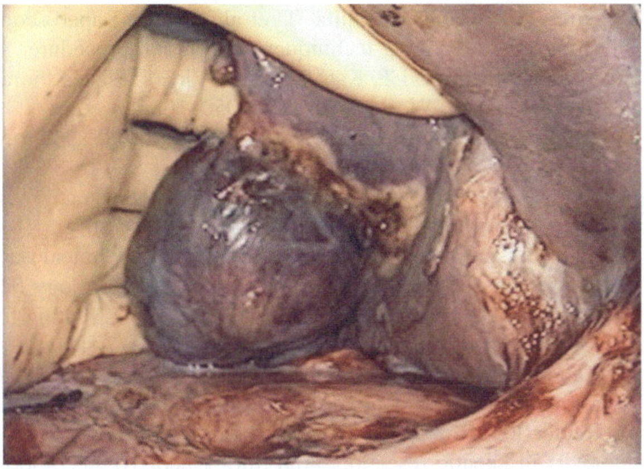

Fig. 14.8 Microwave precoagulation on transection line

which microwave was used during laparoscopic liver resection [11]. Because HCC is frequently accompanied by chronic liver disease, a modality for transection in the cirrhotic liver is required. Using the above-mentioned surgical technique, LH for HCC was successful and resulted in long-term outcomes that were identical to those of open conventional hepatectomy [3]. Reuter et al. also found that microwave energy was safe and effective for precoagulation in both open and laparoscopic technique. It has achieved good hemostasis during hepatic resection [12]. However, vessel injury by insertion of needle antenna into the liver parenchyma may cause complications (i.e., bile leakage, biliary stricture, liver abscess, or aneurysm); careful exploration using intraoperative ultrasound should be taken to avoid injury to vessels. In particular, it should not be applied beside the hepatic hilum.

14.4 Conclusions

Although laparoscopic liver resection requires careful selection of patients and instrumentation, use of microwave tissue coagulation could contribute to safe laparoscopic liver surgery.

References

1. Buell JF, Cherqui D, Geller DA et al. (2009) The international position on laparoscopic liver surgery: the Louisville Statement, 2008. Ann Surg 250:825–830
2. Kaneko H, Otsuka Y, Tsuchiya M et al. (2008) Application of devices for safe laparoscopic hepatectomy. HPB 10:219–224
3. Kaneko H, Tsuchiya M, Otsuka Y et al. (2009) Laparoscopic hepatectomy for hepatocellular carcinoma in cirrhotic patients. J Hepatobiliary Pancreat Surg 16:433–438
4. Koffron A, Auffenberg G, Kung R et al. (2007) Evaluation of 300 minimally invasive liver resections at a single institution: less is more. Ann Surg 246:385–394

5. Nitta H, Sasaki A, Fujita T et al. (2010) Laparoscopy-assisted major liver resections employing a hanging technique: the original procedure. Ann Surg 251:450–453
6. Murakami M, Aoki T, Kato T (2011) Video-assisted thoracoscopic surgery: hepatectomy for liver neoplasm. World J Surg 35:1050–1054
7. Tabuse K, Katsumi M, Kobayashi Y et al. (1985) Microwave surgery: hepatectomy using a microwave tissue coagulator. World J Surg 9:136–143
8. Ryu M, Watanabe K, Yamamoto H (1998) Hepatectomy with microwave tissue coagulation for hepatocellular carcinoma. J Hep Bil Pancr Surg 5:184–191
9. Satoi S, Kamiyama Y, Matsui Y et al. (2005) Clinical outcome of 214 liver resections using microwave tissue coagulation. Hepatogastroenterology 52:1180–1185
10. Christian DJ, Khithani A, Jeyarajah DR (2011) Making liver transection even safer: a novel use of microwave technology. Am Surg 77:417–421
11. Kaneko H, Takagi S, Shiba S (1996) Laparoscopic partial hepatectomy and left lateral segmentectomy: technique and results of a clinical series. Surgery 120:468–475
12. Reuter PN, Robert CG, Martin II (2009) Microwave energy as a precoagulative device to assist in hepatic resection. Ann Surg Oncol 16:3057–3063

Laparoscopic Liver Resection Using LPMOD

15

Xiu Jun Cai, Yi Fan Wang and Shu You Peng

The laparoscopic approach has developed greatly in the last 20 years [1–4]. It allows the patient rapid return to daily activity and has been adopted almost worldwide. Laparoscopic hepatectomy is still a difficult and risky procedure and is only performed in a few large institutions in spite of the advantage of minimal invasion. The main reason is that the liver has rich blood supply and hepatic inflow occlusion is difficult to accomplish laparoscopically. Current instruments used in laparoscopic liver resection include ultrasonic knife, LigaSure, linear staple, etc. Our institution began to perform laparoscopic hepatectomy by curettage and aspiration (LHCA) using a proven version of Peng's multifunctional operative dissector (PMOD), named the laparoscopic Peng's multifunctional operative dissector (LPMOD) (Fig. 15.1).

Electronic Supplementary Material The online version of this article (doi:10.1007/978-88-470-2622-3_15) contains supplementary material which is available to authorized users.

X. J. Cai · Y. F. Wang
Department of Surgery, Sir Run Run Shaw Hospital, Zhejiang University, 3 East Qinchun Road, Hangzhou, 310016 Zhejiang, People's Republic of China
e-mail: cxjzu@hotmail.com

Y. F. Wang
e-mail: anwyf@163.com

S. Y. Peng (✉)
Department of Surgery, Sir Run Run Shaw Hospital, Zhejiang University, Second Affiliated Hospital of Zhejiang University, 88 Jiefang Road, Hangzhou, 310009 Zhejiang, People's Republic of China
e-mail: zrwkpsy@zju.edu.cn

I. Di Carlo (ed.), *Open, Laparoscopic and Robotic Hepatic Transection*,
DOI: 10.1007/978-88-470-2622-3_15,

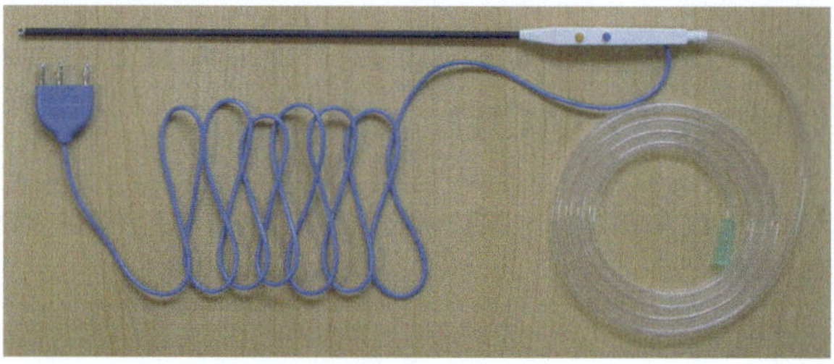

Fig. 15.1 Laparoscopic Peng's multifunctional operative dissector (LPMOD)

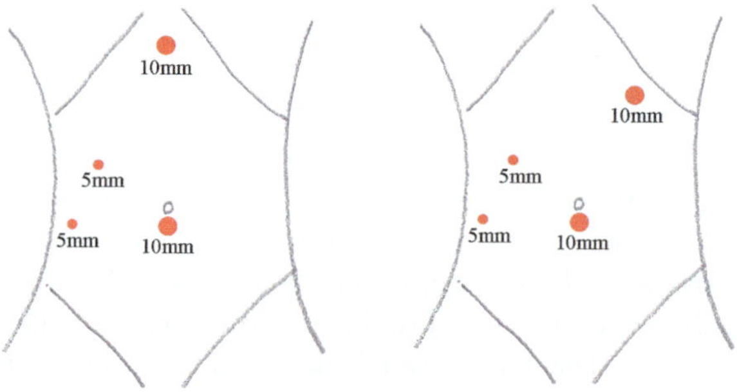

Fig. 15.2 Entry positions for right liver lesion (*right*) and for left liver lesion (*left*)

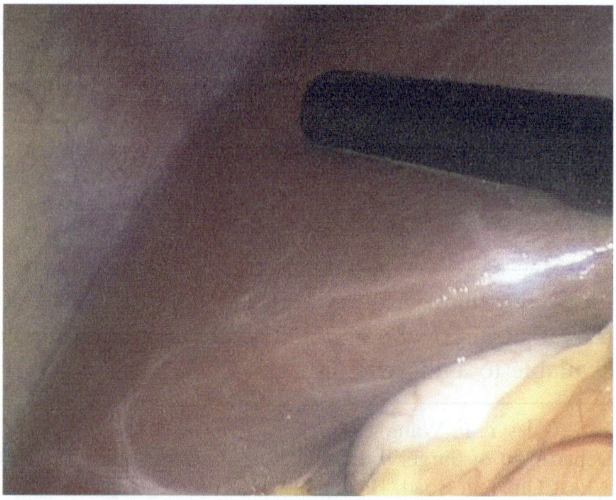

Fig. 15.3 Ultrasound was applied to locate lesions

15.1 Instrument

Compared with PMOD, the length of the stalk of the LPMOD was extended to fit laparoscopic procedure while retaining all the functions of the PMOD. Like the PMOD, the enhanced instrument can be used for blunt dissection, aspiration and irrigation, cutting, and electric coagulation, all at the same time. Intrahepatic ducts and vessels can be safely bluntly dissected with it. Furthermore, the

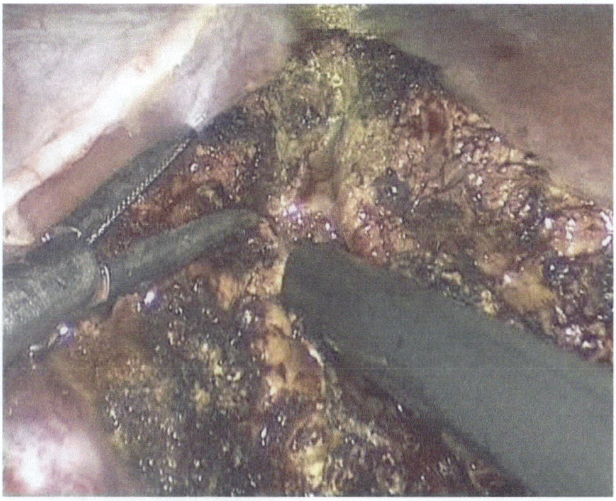

Fig. 15.4 Liver parenchyma was bluntly dissected

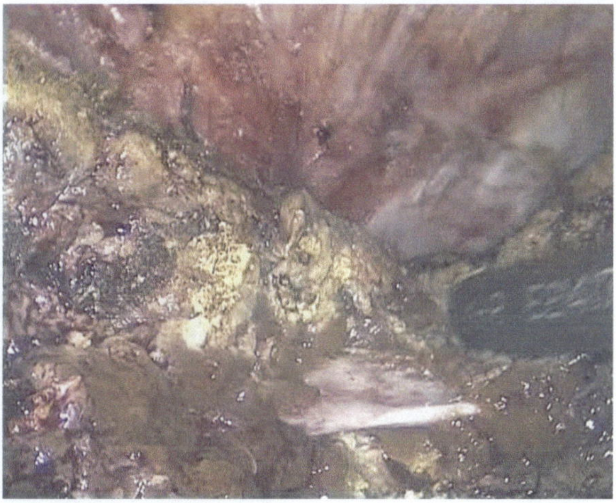

Fig. 15.5 Vessels were conserved by blunt dissection

LPMOD is not as expensive as other instruments, such as ultrasonic knife and LigaSure, for laparoscopic hepatectomy. The advantage of LPMOD over other instruments is that LPMOD combines the functions of anatomical transection and hemostasis.

15.2 Procedure

A totally laparoscopic approach was performed under general anesthesia. Three surgeons were required for this operation: two of them in charge of liver transection, and the third assigned to control the aspirator by clamping the aspiration tube with a forceps. Patients were placed in supine position, after which

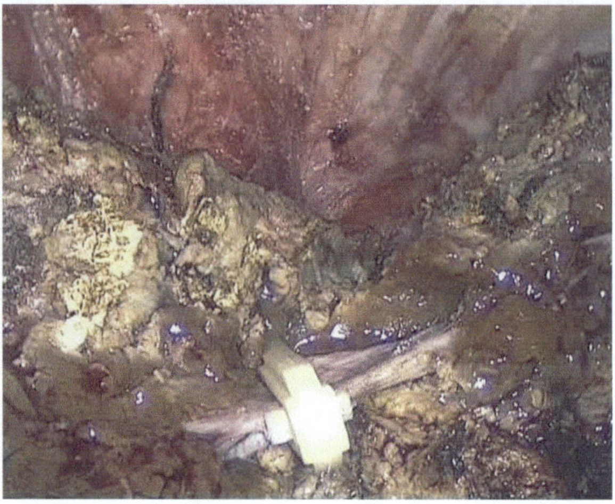
Fig. 15.6 A dissected vessel was freed and clamped

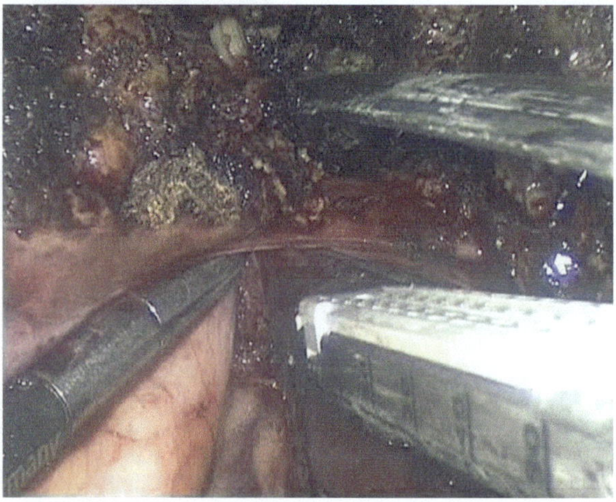
Fig. 15.7 Larger vessels were divided by linear staple

pneumoperitoneum was established and CO_2 gas pressure was set at 14 mmHg. Four incisions were made (Fig. 15.2): One 10-mm port for the laparoscope was placed below the umbilicus; The other 10-mm port for LPMOD for surgery was placed under the xiphoid process or under left costal margin for right or left liver lesion, respectively; Two 5-mm ports were placed in the right mid-abdomen for the assistant [5–7].

The abdominal cavity was inspected first, and lesions were located by laparoscopic ultrasound (Fig. 15.3). The transaction line was marked on the liver surface based on perioperative imaging and intraoperative ultrasound. With the LPMOD, the liver capsule was cut open, the liver parenchyma was bluntly dissected (Fig. 15.4), and the transection plane was coagulated to control minor bleeding. Liver fragments, blood, and smoke were aspirated by LPMOD simultaneously. By using blunt dissection, duct structures could be safely conserved (Fig. 15.5) and freed (Fig. 15.6), then clamped and divided. Endo-GIA may be applied to ducts larger than 10 mm in diameter (Fig. 15.7). This maneuver was repeated until the liver was completely transected. A 3–5 cm laparotomy incision was made by extending a 5-cm laparoscopic entire, and the entire specimen was removed in a plastic bag.

For dissection of liver parenchyma, the liver capsule was opened and the superficial liver parenchyma up to 5 mm in depth was cut by the tip of the LPMOD, after which the tip was used for blunt dissection of the liver parenchyma. Liver fragments were aspirated repeatedly to make the surgical field clear. While transecting liver parenchyma, the tenacity of vessels and the firmness of intrahepatic ducts make their identification easy: the operator can feel resistance when encountering vessels or hepatic ducts. Operator should apply curettage and dissection parallel to those structures until a 1-cm segment is freed, then clamp and transect the vessels and hepatic ducts. In general, small vessels or ducts can be ligated with 10-mm titanium clips or with 12 mm absorbable ligating clips. Structures larger than 10 mm can be divided with a linear stapler. With this technique, there is little blood loss and the insufflated gas has much less chance to get into blood circulation.

References

1. Koffron AJ, Auffenberg G, Kung R, Abecassis M (2007) Evaluation of 300 minimally invasive liver resections at a single institution: less is more. Ann Surg 246(3):385–392, discussion 392–394
2. Nguyen KT, Gamblin TC, Geller DA (2009) World review of laparoscopic liver resection-2,804 patients. Ann Surg 250(5):831–841 (Review)
3. Buell JF, Cherqui D, Geller DA, O'Rourke N, Iannitti D, Dagher I, Koffron AJ, Thomas M, Gayet B, Han HS, Wakabayashi G, Belli G, Kaneko H, Ker CG, Scatton O, Laurent A, Abdalla EK, Chaudhury P, Dutson E, Gamblin C, D'Angelica M, Nagorney D, Testa G, Labow D, Manas D, Poon RT, Nelson H, Martin R, Clary B, Pinson WC, Martinie J, Vauthey JN, Goldstein R, Roayaie S, Barlet D, Espat J, Abecassis M, Rees M, Fong Y, McMasters KM, Broelsch C, Busuttil R, Belghiti J, Strasberg S, Chari RS, World Consensus Conference on Laparoscopic Surgery (2009) The international position on laparoscopic liver surgery: the Louisville Statement, 2008. Ann Surg 250(5):825–830
4. Bryant R, Laurent A, Tayar C, Cherqui D (2009) Laparoscopic liver resection-understanding its role in current practice: the Henri Mondor Hospital experience. Ann Surg 250(1):103–111
5. Cai XJ, Yu H, Liang X, Wang YF, Zheng XY, Huang DY, Peng SY (2006) Laparoscopic hepatectomy by curettage and aspiration. Experiences of 62 cases. Surg Endosc 20(10): 1531–1535
6. Cai XJ, Wang YF, Liang YL, Yu H, Liang X (2009) Laparoscopic left hemihepatectomy: a safety and feasibility study of 19 cases. Surg Endosc 23(11):2556–2562
7. Cai X, Wang Y, Yu H, Liang X, Peng S (2007) Laparoscopic hepatectomy for hepatolithiasis: a feasibility and safety study in 29 patients. Surg Endosc 21(7):1074–1078

Laparoscopic Hepatic Transection Using Radiofrequency Monopolar Devices

16

Isidoro Di Carlo and Adriana Toro

16.1 Introduction

It is now recognized that laparoscopic liver resection (LLR) can be performed for both benign and malignant conditions with safety and outcomes comparable to the open approach [1].

In laparoscopic surgery, hepatic transection must be performed using a device and is more technically demanding and potentially more hazardous than in open surgery. For this reason, precise coagulation of hepatic parenchyma and its small vessels is the correct method for identification of the main structures and performance of safe resection.

The Sealing Hook (SH) (Salient Endo SH 3.0) and Monopolar Floating Ball (FB) (Salient Endo FB 3.0) (Salient Surgical Technologies, Dover, NH, USA) are two devices designed for coagulation and/or parenchymal transection of the liver using radiofrequency-based technology.

The aim of this chapter is to describe these devices for laparoscopic surgery and related technique.

I. Di Carlo (✉) · A. Toro
Department of Surgical Sciences, Organ Transplantation and Advanced Technologies, University of Catania, Cannizzaro Hospital, Via Messina, 829, 95126 Catania, Italy
e-mail: idicarlo@unict.it

A. Toro
e-mail: atoroct@gmail.com

I. Di Carlo (ed.), *Open, Laparoscopic and Robotic Hepatic Transection*,
DOI: 10.1007/978-88-470-2622-3_16,

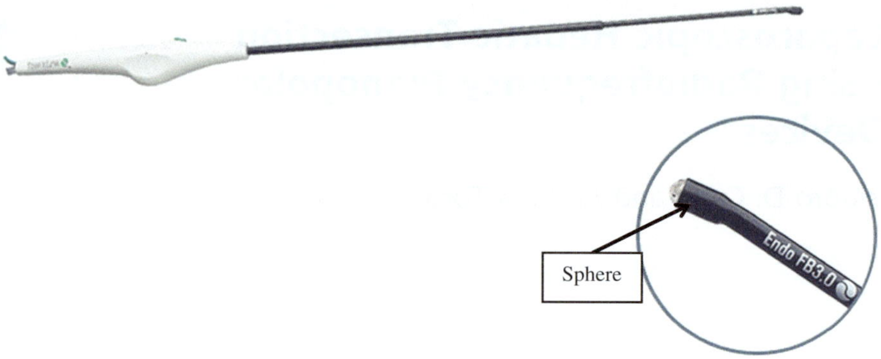

Fig. 16.1 FB; the tip as a "sphere" limits the use of this device

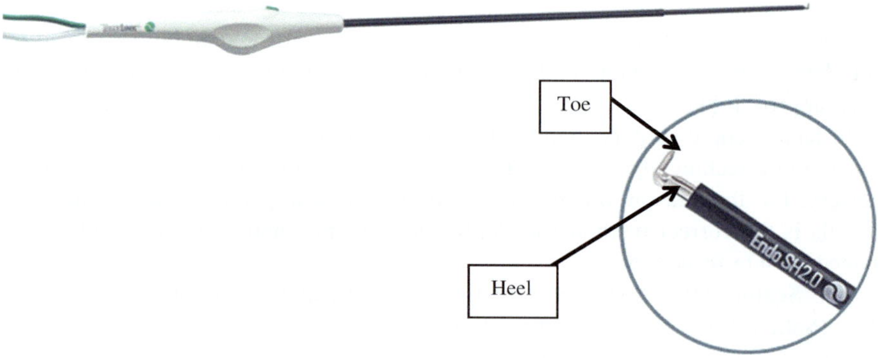

Fig. 16.2 The special structure of the tip gives the instrument more possibilities of use

16.2 Device Description

The FB (Fig. 16.1) and SH (Fig. 16.2) are sterile, single-use electrosurgery devices intended to be used in conjunction with an electrosurgical generator for delivery of radiofrequency (RF) current and saline, for hemostatic sealing and coagulation of soft tissue at the operative site.

Both devices have a proximal and a distal end, comprising: a handle; a button in the middle of superior part of the handle; a shaft extending from the handle, the shaft supporting an electrode tip in rigid relation to the handle and having a distal end; a fluid passage being connectable to a fluid source.

The electrode tip comprises a single metal contact element providing an electrode having a distal portion and a proximal portion, the distal portion of the electrode extending distally beyond the distal end of the shaft and the proximal portion of the electrode being contained within the shaft.

The distal portion of the electrode differs between the FB and SH. In the former, the tip is circumferential like a "sphere" (Fig. 16.1). In the SH there is a hook with a "heel" and a "toe" (Fig. 16.2).

The device is connected to a standard electrocautery unit and to a bag of 0.9% normal saline. The surgeon can activate the device using the button located on the handle and simultaneously manipulate the distal tip during treatment.

Hepatic tissue is gently heated during hepatic resection; tissue collagen, when treated, can seal vascular structures and stroma while simultaneously coagulating the hepatocyte/sinusoid. In most instances, the electrocautery unit is set to 120 W (coagulation) and the saline drip rate to 1 drop/s.

16.3 Technique Description

The surgeon is usually positioned at the foot of the table, with one laparoscope operator to the right and one assistant to the left. The patient is placed in reverse Trendelenburg position. In case of anterior or left liver lesions, the patient is placed supine and rotated about 30° grades to the left. For posterior lesions of the right liver, the patient is placed in left lateral decubitus position, allowing access to the midline. Pneumoperitoneum is controlled electronically to pressure of 10 mmHg.

A 12-mm umbilical port is used for the 30° laparoscope. Additional working ports are placed strategically to optimize the procedure. Port sites are placed in anticipation of open conversion so that the port sites are in line with standard surgical incisions, if needed. The number of trocars used may vary depending on tumor location and surgeon preference. A laparoscopic ultrasound transducer is used to map out the position of the vascular and biliary structures and to demarcate surgical tumor resection margins.

After inspection of the liver by ultrasound, a line of demarcation is provided. This line can be performed using the FB (Fig. 16.3) or SH, momentarily stopping the saline flow. After the Glissonian opening, superficial transection can start. Both devices can be used to precoagulate liver parenchyma.

The activated handle (button pressed) has to be used with gentle pressure on the liver parenchyma combined with rotational movements. Using the FB, after pre-coagulation, another device has to be used to transect the liver parenchyma depending on surgeon preference; in contrast, not only can the SH be used with the "heel" to transect the liver but structures can then be hooked with the "toe" of the device, further coagulated briefly, and then divided by pulling the device, similar to the action of hook cautery during laparoscopic cholecystectomy.

When hepatic transection proceeds deeper into liver parenchyma, larger vessels are encountered; vessels identified and isolated may be treated using a device of choice, due to the fact that neither device (SH or FB) can coagulate and seal vessels of more than 7 mm. Once transection is completed, the SH or FB can be used to achieve hemostasis; in this regard, circular motion provides the best result.

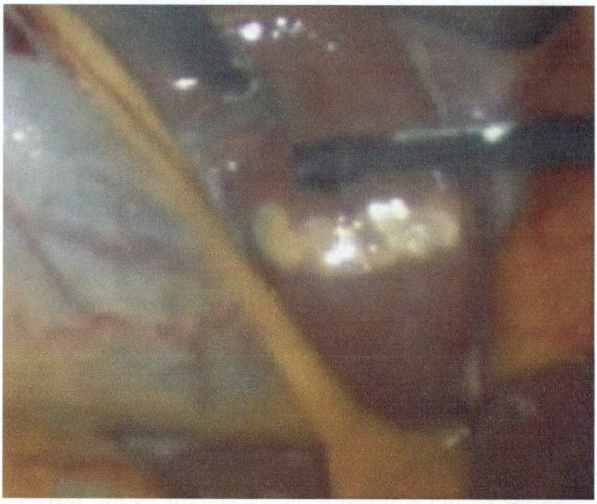

Fig. 16.3 FB can initially provide demarcation of Glisson's surface of liver to be resected

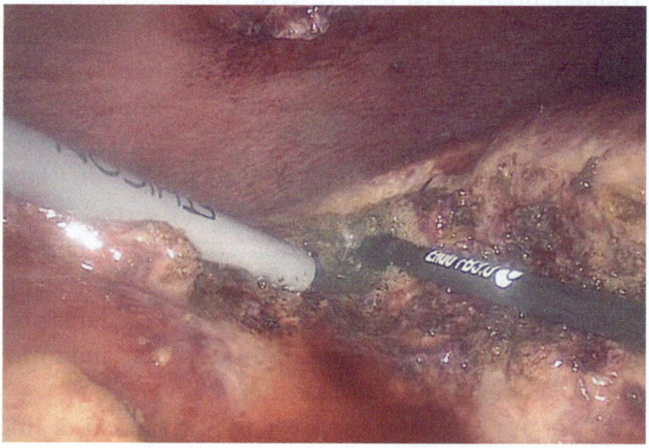

Fig. 16.4 In case of tumoral resection that needs to spare tissue, FB can achieve oncological radicality

In case hepatic resection is not oncologically radical, the FB or SH could induce a pronounced heat-zone area (Fig. 16.4), and possible remaining tumoral cells could be efficiently destroyed [2].

FB and SH should be managed with caution in presence of biliary structure and diaphragm; also, contact with metal objects has to be absolutely avoided due to the possibility of conduction and arcing. Steatotic liver requires more contact with electrocautery working on a lower power setting (around 90 W). In contrast, fibrotic/cirrhotic liver requires less device treatment but with careful dissection because tactile feedback is diminished by the inherent tissue turgor [3].

References

1. Buell JF, Cherqui D, Geller DA, O'Rourke N, Iannitti D, Dagher I, Koffron AJ, Thomas M, Gayet B, Han HS, Wakabayashi G, Belli G, Kaneko H, Ker CG, Scatton O, Laurent A, Abdalla EK, Chaudhury P, Dutson E, Gamblin C, D'Angelica M, Nagorney D, Testa G, Labow D, Manas D, Poon RT, Nelson H, Martin R, Clary B, Pinson WC, Martinie J, Vauthey JN, Goldstein R, Roayaie S, Barlet D, Espat J, Abecassis M, Rees M, Fong Y, McMasters KM, Broelsch C, Busuttil R, Belghiti J, Strasberg S, Chari RS (2009) World consensus conference on laparoscopic surgery. The international position on laparoscopic liver surgery: the Louisville statement, 2008. Ann Surg 250:825–830
2. Kianmanesh R, Ogata S, Paradis V, Sauvanet A, Belghiti J (2008) Heat-zone effect after surface application of dissecting sealer on the "in situ margin" after tumorectomy for liver tumors. J Am Coll Surg 206:1122–1128
3. Koffron AJ, Auffenberg G, Kung R, Abecassis M (2007) Evaluation of 300 minimally invasive liver resections at a single institution: less is more. Ann Surg 246:385–392

Laparoscopic Hepatic Transection Using Habib™ 4X

17

Madhava Pai, Charis Kyriakides, Feng Xi and Nagy A. Habib

17.1 Introduction

The first laparoscopic liver resection (LHR) was reported by Reich et al. in 1991, and the first successful laparoscopic anatomical hepatectomy (segments II and III) was performed in a patient with a benign adenoma in 1996 [1, 2]. Thanks to the significant progress in laparoscopic procedures and the development of new technologies in recent years, laparoscopic liver resection has become a feasible and safe procedure [3, 4]. Excellent results in terms of perioperative morbidity and mortality among patients with good liver function using conventional laparoscopic surgical methods were reported in high-volume centers. Nevertheless, it remains a

Electronic Supplementary Material The online version of this article (doi:10.1007/978-88-470-2622-3_17) contains supplementary material which is available to authorized users.

M. Pai · C. Kyriakides · F. Xi · N. A. Habib (✉)
HPB Surgery, Hammersmith Hospital, Imperial College London,
Du Cane Road, London,
W12 0HS, UK
e-mail: nagy.habib@imperial.ac.uk
M. Pai
e-mail: madhava.pai@imperial.ac.uk

C. Kyriakides
e-mail: Charis.kyriakides@imperial.nhs.uk

F. Xi
e-mail: Feng.xi.cn@gmail.com

I. Di Carlo (ed.), *Open, Laparoscopic and Robotic Hepatic Transection*, DOI: 10.1007/978-88-470-2622-3_17, © Springer-Verlag Italia 2012

technically demanding procedure. Obstacles to laparoscopic liver resection mainly arise from limited access around the liver, a lack of dedicated laparoscopic liver retractors, the absence of tactile feedback for surgeons, the potential catastrophic consequences of injuring major adjacent structures, difficulty in safe parenchymal transection, and bleeding. Among various intra- and postoperative complications, bleeding represents the most serious problem for the surgeon during laparoscopic liver surgery. In spite of the development of various devices designed to minimize blood loss during liver parenchymal transection, hemorrhage is difficult to control laparoscopically, remaining the main cause of conversion to laparotomy [5, 6]. In addition, these devices are usually used in combination with hepatic pedicle clamping to achieve satisfactory intraoperative hemostasis, because none of these techniques is effective in preventing intraoperative bleeding on its own. As a result, consequent ischemia–reperfusion and warm ischemia injury to the liver increase the risk of postoperative liver dysfunction or failure, further compromising the outcome of laparoscopic liver resections. In areas where a considerable part of liver surgery is performed on cirrhotic patients with chronically impaired liver function secondary to chronic hepatitis B virus infection, this issue may become even more significant.

Radiofrequency (RF)-assisted liver surgery is so far the only surgical technique that reduces blood loss while increasing parenchymal sparing, with reduced or even no liver warm ischemia. RF is used to create a plane of coagulative necrosis along the intended line of parenchymal transection in order to reduce blood loss during transection of liver parenchyma. This technique was first reported by Weber et al., who used a monopolar RF ablation device in open hepatic resection [7]. A significant reduction of blood loss was found in patients who underwent liver resection using this device. Further research on the efficiency of RF energy led to the development of a bipolar, handheld, disposable RF device known as the Habib™ 4X, which requires no need for vascular clamping, suturing or clipping. Because of these unique features, its application in laparoscopic surgery offers major advantages. Its successful deployment in open liver surgery has led to the birth of a new device, the Laparoscopic Habib™ 4X (LH4X), for laparoscopic liver resection.

17.2 Device Description

The Laparoscopic Habib™ 4X, consisting of a 2×2 array of needles arranged in a rectangle, uses bipolar RF energy (Fig. 17.1). The LH4X measures 45 cm in length with a protected insulated area, to allow 5 cm length for RF exposure. The device can be introduced via a 10–12-mm laparoscopic port and is connected to a 500-kHz generator (model 1500X; AngioDynamics Inc., Queensbury, NY, USA) which produces up to 250 W of RF power. It allows measurement of the generator output, tissue impedance, temperature, and time of application. The system also includes a pneumatic foot pedal used to activate/deactivate the RF probe. The generator can be run in manual or automatic mode. On connecting the device and switching on the generator, the RF power setting defaults to 125 W; this can be

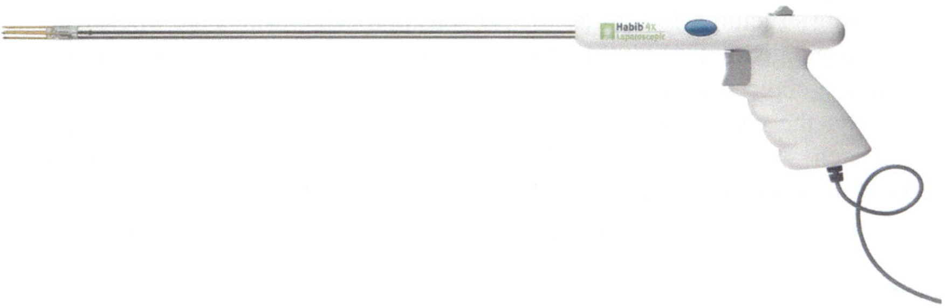

Fig. 17.1 Laparoscopic Habib 4X bipolar radiofrequency device

modified according to user experience and the thermal requirement of the various tissue types.

17.3 Operative Technique

Under general anesthesia, for resections of segments II–V, the patient is placed in supine position. For lesions in segment VI, the patient is placed in left lateral decubitus position, to maximize exposure of the posterolateral aspect of the right lobe. The open technique for creation of pneumoperitoneum is preferred to avoid possible damage to intra-abdominal structures, especially in patients with multiple previous abdominal explorations. Pneumoperitoneum is maintained throughout the procedure on a high flow rate with CO_2 at pressure of 12 mmHg. Three 12-mm and one 5-mm ports are usually sufficient, placed along the subcostal margin depending on the tumor site. Specifically, two 12-mm ports are inserted on one side whereas one 12-mm and one 5-mm port are inserted on the contralateral site. Any perihepatic and peritoneal adhesions related to previous laparotomies are divided to allow full examination of the entire peritoneal cavity for either local recurrence at the site of previous colorectal resection or peritoneal deposits. Laparoscopic intraoperative ultrasound (LIOUS; Aloka Co., Ltd., Tokyo, Japan) is carried out in all patients to obtain further information on the extent of disease and the anatomical relationship between the portal pedicles, hepatic venous branches, and the tumor. The technique of laparoscopic liver resection assisted by LH4X is similar to the previously described open approach. In brief, LH4X is used to produce coagulative necrosis along the line of intended parenchymal transection without vascular clamping of either portal triads or major vessels.

However, some important differences have to be mentioned. Following routine LIOUS examination of the liver prior to starting LH4X-assisted liver resection, the intended transection plane is marked on the surface of the liver with diathermy. Then, the LH4X is inserted first to the most difficult part of the intended plane of transection, in the deepest and farthest areas from the surface of the liver under the guidance of LIOUS. This is to prevent the RF probe and tissue coagulation from interfering with the ultrasonic images, thereby preventing accurate localization of the tumor and its neighboring structures. In contrast to the open approach in which the whole resection line is coagulated before cutting, the liver parenchyma is progressively transected with laparoscopic scissors after each RF application until completion.

Finally, the specimen is extracted whenever possible with an Endobag^{TM} or Endo Catch^{TM} (Covidien, Norwalk, CT, USA) by enlarging a port-site incision or through a suprapubic one. A 20 FG drain (Smiths Medical International Ltd., Hythe, Kent, UK) was routinely placed close to the resection margin.

References

1. Reich H, McGlynn F, DeCaprio J, Budin R (1991) Laparoscopic excision of benign liver lesions. Obstet Gynecol 78:956–958
2. Azagra JS, Goergen M, Gilbart E, Jacobs D (1996) Laparoscopic anatomical (hepatic) left lateral segmentectomy-technical aspects. Surg Endosc 10:758–761
3. Nguyen KT, Gamblin TC, Geller DA (2009) World review of laparoscopic liver resection-2,804 patients. Ann Surg 250:831–841
4. Spencer L, Metcalfe MS, Strickland AD, Elsey EJ, Robertson GS, Lloyd DM (2008) Lessons from laparoscopic liver surgery: a nine-year case series. HPB Surg 2008:458137
5. Belli G, Fantini C, D'Agostino A, Cioffi L, Langella S, Russolillo N, Belli A (2007) Laparoscopic versus open liver resection for hepatocellular carcinoma in patients with histologically proven cirrhosis: short- and middle-term results. Surg Endosc 21:2004–2011
6. Dagher I, Lainas P, Carloni A, Caillard C, Champault A, Smadja C, Franco D (2008) Laparoscopic liver resection for hepatocellular carcinoma. Surg Endosc 22:372–378
7. Weber JC, Navarra G, Jiao LR, Nicholls JP, Jensen SL, Habib NA (2002) New technique for liver resection using heat coagulative necrosis. Ann Surg 236:560–563

Laparoscopic Hepatic Transection Using Stapler and CUSA

18

Francesca Ratti, Federica Cipriani, Marco Catena,
Michele Paganelli and Luca Aldrighetti

18.1 Introduction

Laparoscopic liver surgery has attracted increasing interest in a growing number of hepatobiliary centers since the development of newer laparoscopic instruments and techniques [1].

Postoperative morbidity and mortality for patients undergoing liver resection are closely related to the amount of intraoperative blood loss, the majority of which occurs during transection of liver parenchyma [2]. Many studies in the literature demonstrate that laparoscopy is associated with reduced blood loss and morbidity and that these advantages are even more evident in cirrhotic patients [3–5]; efficient and safe laparoscopic liver transection is dependent on the ability

---

Electronic Supplementary Material The online version of this article (doi:10.1007/978-88-470-2622-3_18) contains supplementary material which is available to authorized users.

F. Ratti (✉) · F. Cipriani · M. Catena · M. Paganelli · L. Aldrighetti
Department of Surgery, Hepatobiliary Surgery Unit, San Raffaele Hospital,
Vita-Salute San Raffaele University, Via Olgettina 60, 20132 Milan MI, Italy
e-mail: ratti.francesca@hsr.it

F. Cipriani
e-mail: cipriani.federica@hsr.it

M. Catena
e-mail: catena.marco@hsr.it

M. Paganelli
e-mail: paganelli.michele@hsr.it

L. Aldrighetti
e-mail: aldrighetti.luca@hsr.it

I. Di Carlo (ed.), *Open, Laparoscopic and Robotic Hepatic Transection*,
DOI: 10.1007/978-88-470-2622-3_18, © Springer-Verlag Italia 2012

to simultaneously address two tasks: parenchymal division and hemostasis [6]. Over the past years, technological advances have led to the development of specific instruments for liver transection, such as the ultrasonic dissector, which has become the standard tool used in many centers in both open and laparoscopic surgery [7, 8]. Recently, stapler devices have been extensively used to address the task of parenchymal transection, in addition to transection of major vessels [9, 10].

18.2 Device Description

18.2.1 Stapler

Endoscopic stapling devices have become increasingly utilized in laparoscopic operations; in laparoscopic liver surgery, linear stapler allows delivery of four rows of staples and to cut between the middle two rows. Their use is reported in both transection of large vessels and parenchymal transection [9, 10]. A wide variety of devices exists, and their evolution is linked to significant improvements in surgical results, with shorter operative time, even if associated with higher costs.

Laparoscopic staplers are longer and thinner than open ones, since they can be housed in 12-mm trocars. The stapler can be assembled quite easily since, after cartridge apposition on the articulated arm of the instrument, it is ready for use; it can be rotated freely, allowing comfortable handling and accurate device placement. Use of vascular staplers is recommended in liver surgery; different sizes and angles of closure are available according to the task to address.

18.2.2 Cavitron Ultrasonic Surgical Aspirator

The CUSA® is a major achievement of modern ultrasonic technology that represents the technical evolution of clamp crushing as used in open surgery. The CUSA handpiece contains a hollow titanium tip which vibrates longitudinally along its axis, driven by a magnetostrictive transducer. The vibration occurs at a medium frequency of 23 kHz and with an adjustable stroke of 0–300 μm. The tip of the device, placed in contact with liver parenchyma, destroys and emulsifies cell membranes, which are irrigated and removed through a built-in suction tube. Since vessels and biliary structures larger than 0.5 mm in diameter and fibrous tissue capsules contain much collagen, they rebound with the ultrasonic vibration waves emitted by the CUSA and are consequently left unimpaired by the procedure. The effectiveness also depends upon the amount of water contained in the tissue, so that CUSA is very effective in healthy liver parenchyma but less in cirrhotic livers [6].

Nowadays, the effectiveness of laparoscopic CUSA is well described, in particular in association with the Harmonic Scalpel, thereby integrating the conventional ultrasonic dissector and ultrasonic coagulating cutter [6].

18.3 Technique Description

Postoperative morbidity and mortality are closely related to the amount of intraoperative blood loss, the majority of which occurs during parenchymal transection [2]. Reduced blood loss is one of the reasons why laparoscopic liver surgery is gradually gaining wider acceptance as treatment of choice for liver lesions [1, 4, 5]. Indeed, efficient and safe laparoscopic liver resection is dependent on the ability to simultaneously address two tasks: parenchymal division and hemostasis. The usefulness and safety of combining the ultrasonic dissector for liver transection and the ultrasonic coagulating cutter for hemostasis in open surgery lead to application of this technique widely also in laparoscopic surgery [6]. Patient positioning and the number of trocars used vary depending on tumor location and surgeon preference. Intraoperative ultrasonography is useful to plan the parenchymal transection line, and the extent of the resection is outlined with electrocautery marks. Superficial liver tissue is generally divided using the ultrasonic coagulating cutter, since, in the absence of large vessels and bile ducts, all peripheral liver parenchyma can be divided, avoiding the risk of bleeding or bile leakage. Then, the ultrasonic dissector is used to fracture hepatocytes along the proposed line of division. The ultrasonic dissector is moved in a "painting"-like motion on the liver surface or along the transection grove. This leaves intact arteries, veins, and bile ducts crossing the line of division, and the uncovered bridging structures are sealed and divided using the ultrasonic coagulating cutter or the bipolar coagulator. Repeated, alternating use of the ultrasonic dissector and the ultrasonic coagulating cutter is continued until resection is complete. The ultrasonic dissector allows clear visualization of structures to avoid damage to important structures and ensures best recognition of all intraparenchymal biliary branches, which may cause bile leaks, abscesses, and sepsis in the postoperative period. Koo et al. [11] reported a significantly higher number of heart air emboli in their CUSA group than in their clamp–crush group; however, none of the patients in either group developed clinical symptoms. The importance of these findings is not clear, and specific reports of this event incidence in laparoscopic surgery do not exist. Anyway, it seems that the reported frequency of embolic events in laparoscopic surgery does not differ significantly from that in laparotomy.

Use of an ultrasonic dissector allows adequate surgical margin with minimal sacrifice of normal liver parenchyma, and the laparoscopic ultrasound evaluation guarantees precise determination of tumor location [6].

A decision on hemostatic technique could be made based on vessel size. Blood vessels up to a few millimeters in diameter are easily coagulated by wet bipolar sealing devices; titanium clip usage is an option to seal larger vessels, even if it should be limited in order to avoid conflict and inadequate closure of vascular stapler. The few larger vessels and portal triads that are encountered are ultrasonically dissected and divided using linear staplers, which are considered beneficial in helping to minimize blood loss and thereby reducing the need for inflow occlusion. Recently, an ultrasound-directed transparenchymal application of vascular staplers to selectively divide major intrahepatic blood vessels before the parenchymal phase of liver resection has been shown to minimize blood loss, warm ischemia time, and operative time [7].

Caution has to be applied not to narrow the hepatic duct confluence, especially during right or left hepatectomy for a large tumor encroaching on the liver hilum, which leaves little room for application of the stapler.

In the literature, use of stapler devices to perform parenchymal transection is also reported, especially in laparoscopy; this technique has been mainly applied to left lateral sectionectomy and to pedunculated tumor, as long as it is possible to insert the stapler into the hepatic parenchyma planned for resection [8–10, 12]. One problem associated with stapler use for liver transection is increased risk of bile leak, since the stapler is not very effective in sealing small bile ducts. The crushing effect of vascular staplers on hepatic parenchyma is similar to that of the finger crushing technique as used in open surgery; to avoid unsatisfactory hemostasis, at the end of transection, pneumoperitoneum should be reduced to reveal hidden bleeding sites.

As clear data for comparison of various liver transection techniques are lacking in laparoscopic surgery, currently the choice of technique is often based on individual surgeon preference. At the authors' center, stapler use for parenchymal transection is reserved for selected cases, since CUSA dissection allows better visualization of structures and hemostatic control, leading to better postoperative outcome [13].

Further randomized trials should be performed to compare different liver transection techniques, not only regarding their efficacy in reducing blood loss and safety, but also to evaluate their relative cost-effectiveness.

References

1. Pulitanò C, Aldrighetti L (2008) The current role of laparoscopic liver resection for the treatment of liver tumors. Natl Clin Pract Gastroenterol Hepatol 5:648–654
2. Delis SG, Madariaga J, Bakoyiannis A, Dervenis Ch (2007) Current role of bloodless liver resection. World J Gastroenterol 13:826–829
3. Zhou YM, Shao WY, Zhao YF, Xu DH, Li B (2011) Meta-analysis of laparoscopic versus open resection for hepatocellular carcinoma. Dig Dis Sci 56:1937–1943
4. Pulitanò C, Catena M, Arru M, Guzzetti E, Comotti L, Ferla G, Aldrighetti L (2008) Laparoscopic liver resection without portal clamping: a prospective evaluation. Surg Endosc 22:2196–2200
5. Aldrighetti L, Guzzetti E, Pulitanò C, Cipriani F, Catena M, Paganelli M, Ferla G (2010) Case-matched analysis of totally laparoscopic versus open liver resection for HCC: short and middle term results. J Surg Oncol 102:82–86
6. Aldrighetti L, Pulitanò C, Arru M, Catena M, Guzzetti E, Casati M, Ferla G (2008) Ultrasonic-mediated laparoscopic liver transection. Am J Surg 195:270–272
7. Poon RTP (2007) Current techniques of liver transection. HPB 9:166–173
8. Kaneko H, Otsuka Y, Tsuchiya M, Tamura A, Katagiri T, Yamazaki K (2008) Application of devices for safe laparoscopic hepatectomy. HPB 10:219–224

9. Gumbs AA, Gayet B, Gagner M (2008) Laparoscopic liver resection: when to use the laparoscopic stapler device. HPB 10:296–303
10. Saidi RF, Ahad A, Escobar R, Nalbantoglu I, Adsay V, Jacobs MJ (2007) Comparison between staple and vessel sealing device for parenchymal transection in laparoscopic liver surgery in a swine model. HPB 9:440–443
11. Koo BN, Kil HK, Choi JS, Kim JY, Chun DH, Hong YW (2005) Hepatic resection by the Cavitron Ultrasonic Surgical Aspirator increases the incidence and severity of air embolism. Anesth Analg 101:966–970
12. Aldrighetti L, Pulitanò C, Catena M, Arru M, Guzzetti E, Casati M, Comotti L, Ferla G (2008) A prospective evaluation of laparoscopic versus open left lateral hepatic sectionectomy. J Gastrointest Surg 12:457–462
13. Pamecha V, Gurusamy KS, Sharma D, Davidson BR (2009) Techniques for liver parenchymal transection: a meta-analysis of randomized controlled trials. HPB 11:275–281

Laparoscopic Hepatic Transection Using Ultrasonic Scalpel and Bipolar Forceps

19

Noah B. Zuker and Brice Gayet

19.1 Introduction

The laparoscopic approach to complex disorders of the liver may be extremely useful for enhancing visualization and dissection. As technological advancements lead to more effective tools for laparoscopy, safe and rapid division of liver parenchyma using various techniques has become routine. Ultrasonic dissection is an invaluable tool for dissection and sealing of small to medium-sized vessels during open and laparoscopic procedures. Coupling this rapid modality of cutting tissue with a clamp that is both agile and elegant in the application of electrocautery and retraction leads to efficient and hemostatic procedures.

19.2 Device Description

Ultrasonic scalpel dissection may be employed with hand activation or foot pedal activation. Rotation by 180° of the device head with a gently curved blade facilitates accurate placement. The device typically has two modes of application:

Electronic Supplementary Material The online version of this article (doi:10.1007/978-88-470-2622-3_19) contains supplementary material which is available to authorized users.

N. B. Zuker · B. Gayet (✉)
Département de Pathologie Digestive, L'Institut Mutualiste Monsouris,
42 Boulevard Jourdan, 75674 Cedex 14, Paris, France
e-mail: Brice.gayet@imm.fr

N. B. Zuker
e-mail: noahzuker@gmail.com

I. Di Carlo (ed.), *Open, Laparoscopic and Robotic Hepatic Transection*,
DOI: 10.1007/978-88-470-2622-3_19, © Springer-Verlag Italia 2012

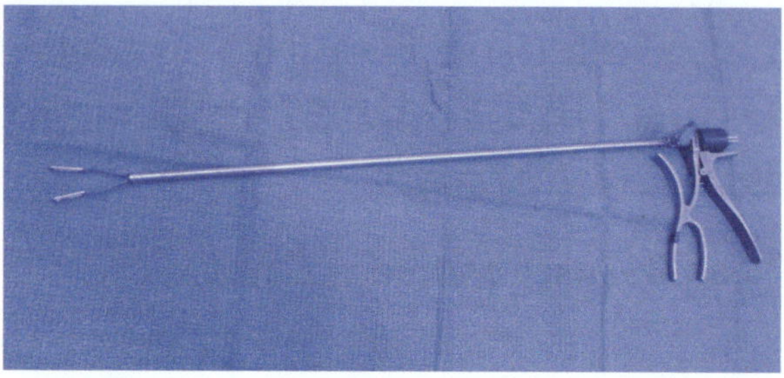

Fig. 19.1 Bipolar forceps

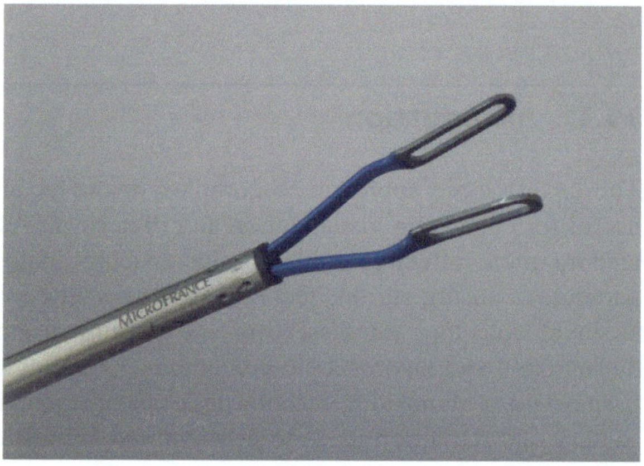

Fig. 19.2 Bipolar forceps detail

slow and fast. Fast cutting may be employed on nonvascular tissue such as adhesions or Glisson's capsule of the liver. Slow coagulation is well suited for division of hepatic parenchyma and small to medium-sized vessels or ducts. Sealing of tubular structures is accomplished by adhering to manufacturer-recommended techniques.

Various handle lengths may be used to accommodate patient body habitus. Typical instruments fit through a 5-mm trocar. The ultrasonic scalpel is most useful for treatment of liver tissue that is relatively normal. For patients with cirrhotic liver, bipolar diathermy devices may be a more secure method to achieve parenchymal transection with superior hemostasis [1]. Ultrasonic scalpel and bipolar coagulation systems have been demonstrated to have no difference in intracorporeal thermal spread [2].

Bipolar forceps (Microfrance™; Medtronic, France) developed specifically for intra-abdominal surgery are a valuable adjunctive tool for clamp dissection, retraction, and bipolar energy application for coagulation (Figs. 19.1, 19.2). Multiple styles of bipolar forceps are modular and adaptable to surgeon preference. Typical design employs an insulated tube that fits through a 5-mm trocar. Pedal activation is used for bipolar force application. Fenestrated forceps provide a wide grasping and retracting surface, and also tend to minimize tissue sticking.

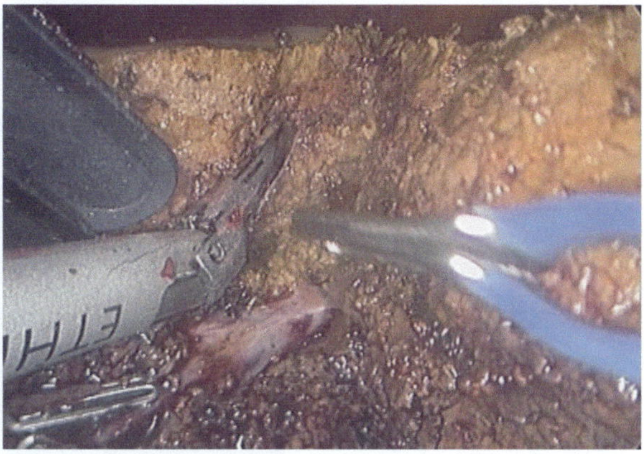

Fig. 19.3 Liver parenchyma with dissecting instrument around the middle hepatic vein

The laparoscopic version is similar to the open surgical forceps; however, the open instrument has a saline irrigation channel that keeps the tips clean for consistent use. During the laparoscopic procedure, surgical technical assistance is required to maintain optimal performance during the course of each operation, because the laparoscopic bipolar clamp lacks an irrigating function. Two sets of forceps must be switched out to provide efficient functioning throughout the course of the operation. We feel that bipolar energy application is the safest and most effective modality for tissue coagulation during complex laparoscopy.

19.3 Description of Technique

Standard surgical principles and techniques are used to provide adequate exposure and traction. Intraoperative ultrasound is always employed to define liver anatomy [3]. The patient is maintained with low CVP to minimize bleeding. This is confirmed by noting the physical characteristics of the inferior vena cava [4]. A smoke evacuator system is employed to optimize visualization. Glisson's capsule is punctured and grasped with the ultrasonic shears on fast cut mode. A push technique may be used to divide the capsule along the resection line. Typically, the liver has few vessels in the most superficial layer; however, ultrasonic coagulation effect requires patience for maximum efficacy. The blade is introduced into the parenchyma while activating the slow cut mode. The jaws are carefully and slowly approximated according to the "give" of the parenchymal tissue sensed by the surgeon's hand. This allows smaller structures to be effectively sealed (Fig. 19.3).

The surgeon employs two-handed dissection with the dissector in the dominant hand and bipolar forceps for retraction. Bipolar forceps are well suited to holding the liver open for further dissection and immediate control via pressure or coagulation. A second pair of bipolar forceps is maintained clean and ready for use when the device becomes encrusted with debris. As larger structures are encountered,

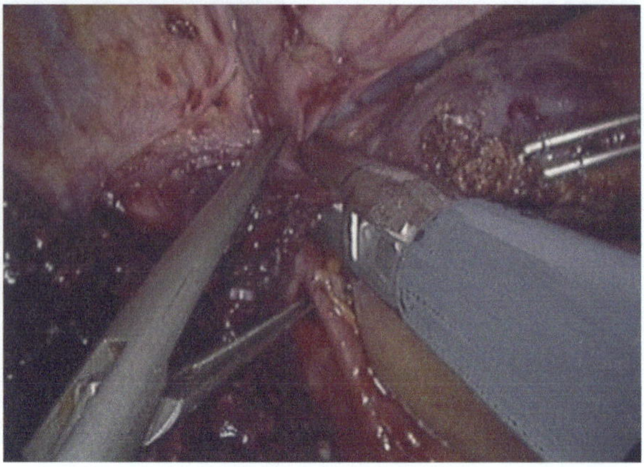

Fig. 19.4 Stapling the left hepatic vein with vascular clamp available

circumferential dissection for control is very important to avoid significant hemorrhage. The ultrasonic active blade may be used in a short-stroke, back-and-forth motion. In this manner it acts similarly to the Cavitron ultrasonic dissector (CUSA^{TM}; Radionics, Burlington, MA, USA) without irrigation of the field or loss of pneumoperitoneum [1]. The blade can be used to gently dissect parenchymal tissue from the vasculature. An ultrasonic device that is inactive on the open edge is ideal for this dissection, and prevents backcutting of tissue that is not enclosed within the jaws. A right-angled clamp completes circumferential dissection. Appropriately sized vessels are coagulated with bipolar cautery and may be clipped and ligated with scissors or ultrasonic scalpel. Very large vessels may require endoscopic stapling. A large vascular clamp (Fig. 19.4) is introduced into the abdomen during stapling of hepatic veins to avoid uncontrollable bleeding [5].

Regarding postoperative bile leakage from the liver cut surface, sealing the tissue with bipolar cautery after division with ultrasonic scalpel has resulted in no postoperative bile leaks. In difficult or complex cases, absorbable hemostatic glue (Tachosil^{TM}; Nycomed, Austria) is applied to the cut surface of the liver as an adjunctive measure. To examine the liver surface, air may be injected into the biliary system to confirm that the system is intact and to detect bile leaks. This technique may be repeated multiple times after suture repair. Bile leak is evidenced by bubbles appearing at the site of the lesion. Examination of liver perfusion and biliary system may be carried out with a near-infrared light camera (Olympus, Japan) after injection of indocyanine green dye. Bile leak appears as a fluorescent pool of bile (Video; Fig. 19.5) easily identified by indocyanine fluorescence after being sequestered in bile [6]. Suture repair is accomplished laparoscopically.

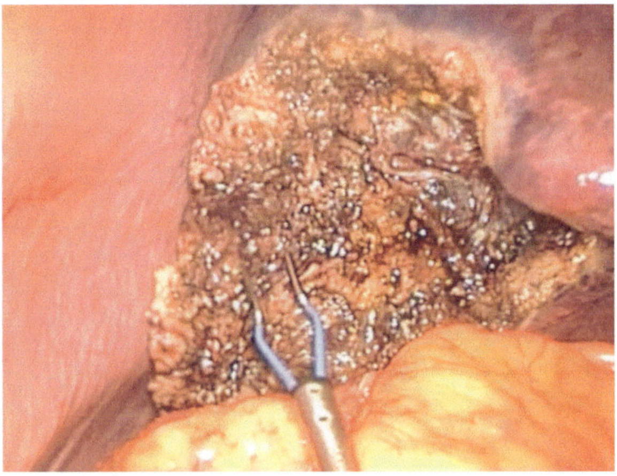

Fig. 19.5 Video diagnosis of bile leak with near-infrared light and indocyanine green. Refer to the video attached within, for further reference

19.4 Conclusions

The combination of two-handed technique with bipolar cautery forceps and the ultrasonic scalpel device allows for efficient parenchymal transection with appropriate control of bleeding vessels and biliary structures. Dissection is accurate and maximizes surgeon capabilities.

References

1. Gumbs AA, Gayet B, Gagner M (2008) Laparoscopic liver resection: when to use the laparoscopic stapler device. HPB 10:296–303
2. Harold KL, Pollinger H, Mathews BD, Kercher KW, Sing RF, Heniford BT (2003) Comparison of ultrasonicultrasonic energy bipolar thermal energy, and vascular clips for the hemostasis of small-, medium-, and large-sized arteries. Surg Endosc 17:1228–1230
3. Hanna SS, Nam R, Leonhardt C (1996) Liver resection by ultrasonic dissection and intraoperative ultrasonography. HPB Surg 9:121–128
4. Gayet B, Cavaliere D, Vibert E, Perniceni T, Levard H, Denet C, Christidis C, Blain A, Mal F (2007) Totally laparoscopic right hepatectomy. Am J Surg 194:685–689
5. Gumbs AA, Bar-Zakai B, Gayet B (2008) Totally laparoscopic extended left hepatectomy. J Gastrointest Surg 12:1152
6. Ishizawa T, Tamura S, Masuda K, Aoki T, Hasegawa K, Imamura H, Beck Y, Kokudo N (2009) Intraoperative fluorescent cholangiography using indocyanine green: a biliary road map for safe surgery. JACS 208:e1–e4

Laparoscopic Hepatic Transection Using an Ultrasonically Activated Device

20

Luigi Cioffi, Andrea Belli, Paolo Limongelli, Gianluca Russo,
Alberto D'Agostino, Corrado Fantini and Giulio Belli

20.1 Introduction

The introduction of new technological devices for efficient and fast hemostatic control during parenchymal transection has greatly enhanced the diffusion and safety of the laparoscopic approach in the field of liver surgery. Among the wide panorama of available devices, the ultrasonically activated device (USAD) in our experience of laparoscopic liver surgery was revealed to be a useful tool in both the dissection and parenchymal transection phases.

20.2 Device Description

The USAD is composed of a generator emitting high-frequency alternating electric current connected to a single-use handpiece containing an acoustic transducer triggering vibration caused by high-frequency electrical energy. The handpiece has an ergonomic and contoured handle with a hook trigger and two power activation buttons. A rotational knob is also present to adapt the bites of the instrument's curved blade to the different needs of surgical dissection.

Electronic Supplementary Material The online version of this article (doi:10.1007/978-88-470-2622-3_20) contains supplementary material which is available to authorized users.

G. Belli (✉)
Department of General and Hepato-Pancreato-Biliary Surgery,
S.M. Loreto Nuovo Hospital, Via Cimarosa 2/A, 80127 Naples, Italy
e-mail: chirurgia.loretonuovo@tin.it

I. Di Carlo (ed.), *Open, Laparoscopic and Robotic Hepatic Transection*,
DOI: 10.1007/978-88-470-2622-3_20, © Springer-Verlag Italia 2012

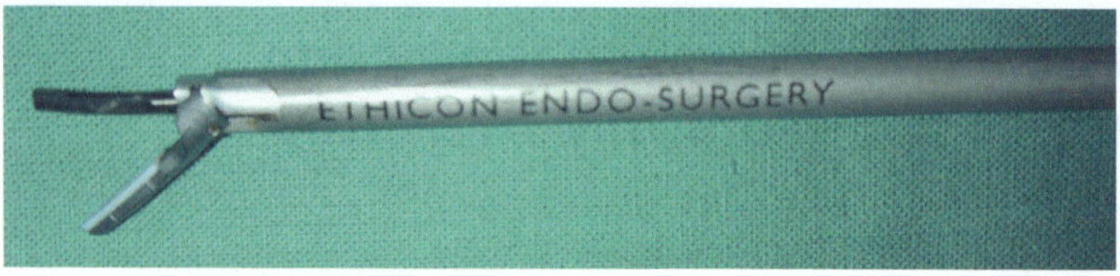

Fig. 20.1 HARMONIC ACE® curved shears with jaw and curved blade enable precise dissection, sealing, and transection near vital structures and of vessels ≤5 mm and lymphatics

The single-use shear consists of an upper anvil and an active lower blade which vibrates longitudinally at a harmonic frequency of 55,000 Hz (Fig. 20.1).

The energy liberated as an ultrasound wave is applied directly to the tissue, thus accomplishing the triple effect of cavitation, coagulation, and cutting. The ultrasonic vibration energy acts by severing hydrogen links, which results in alteration of protein structures, intercellular dissection, and low-temperature vaporization of intra- and extracellular water and hence section of the tissue. The local action of the instrument leads to formation of a protein coagulum and makes the tissue fragile enough to be dissected. The coagulating and sealing power of the instrument allows efficient management of vessels and lymphatics up to 5 mm. The lateral spread of the energy is estimated to be approximately 500 μm, thus minimizing lateral thermal tissue damage for safer dissection near vital structures, which is particularly useful for sealing and cutting small intraparenchymal venous branches (without need for multiple clips) or to dissect the main anatomical structures of the hepatoduodenal ligament.

20.3 Technique Description

All operations were carried out under general anesthesia and controlled CVP maintained at less than 5 mmHg. Patients were placed in the "French" position with the primary surgeon positioned between the legs and one assistant on each side. For lesions located in segments II–III–IV–V we used Lloyd–Davis position, whereas in the case of lesions in right lateral segments we preferred moderate left-lateral decubitus. With an open technique (in order to preserve the umbilical vein), continuous CO_2 pneumoperitoneum was induced at pressure <12 mmHg to prevent the risk of gas embolism. Usually we used a four- or five-trocar configuration. A 12-mm port at the umbilicus housed a 30° video camera. The other trocars were positioned according to the location of the liver lesion (usually along a semicircular line with the concavity facing the right subcostal margin), also including a 5–12-mm port to allow easier instrument exchange, provide the opportunity to use the USAD with both the right and left hand, and facilitate introduction of endostaplers.

A standard diagnostic and staging laparoscopy was performed, and the liver was examined using laparoscopic ultrasonography (BK Medical, San Francisco, USA) (Fig. 20.1) to assess the stage of the disease and evaluate resectability. In

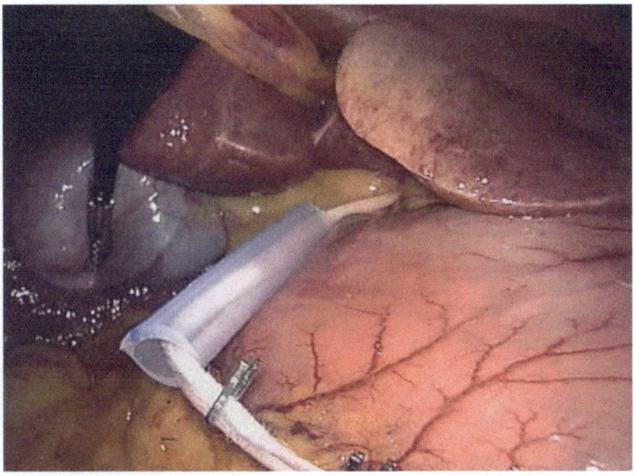

Fig. 20.2 Tape passed around the foramen of Winslow around the porta hepatis to surround the hepatoduodenal pedicle

some cases, round ligament transection was spared. In this way it is possible to preserve the umbilical vein, an important route of collateral blood flow in cirrhotic patients. In some cases, the falciform ligament was incised to allow more comfortable management of the camera and instruments. Once resection had been decided, liver mobilization is accomplished according to planned liver resection; hepatogastric ligament is opened to inspect the Winslow foramen and place a tourniquet around the hepato-duodenal ligament to perform the Pringle maneuver, if necessary (Fig. 20.2). Hepatic arterial and portal vein branches are tied during formal hepatectomy, whilst hepatic veins are generally sutured, generally with an intrahepatic approach using a vascular stapler. When resection regards one or more liver segment(s), the respective portal branches are tied and cut or stapled.

Parenchymal transection starts under ultrasound guidance, incising the liver capsule with electric hook to outline the surgical plane. USAD is employed to divide the liver tissue using medium energy at amplifier setting 3 and in blunt fashion (Fig. 20.3).

The clamping tip of the USAD is employed to grasp and dissect tissues without the need for multiple instrument exchanges. The curved blade of the instrument, easily adaptable to the often curved resection line, especially in case of nonanatomic resections, has a blunt nose for spot coagulation and fine dissection and a cutting edge useful for tissue scoring (drawing of the resection line on the Glisson capsule) or back-cutting.

In case of major hepatectomies or atypical resection, approximately the first 3 cm of liver thickness can be very safely managed by repeated bites of the USAD without causing bleeding, important bile leakage, or trauma because of the absence of large vessels and bile ducts (Fig. 20.4).

Deep in the liver, it is important to activate the USAD only if the tip of the instrument is well visible, thus avoiding injury to small venous branches tributaries of the main hepatic veins. More caution must be paid when dissecting and isolating larger vascular and biliary structures, which have to be separated from hepatic

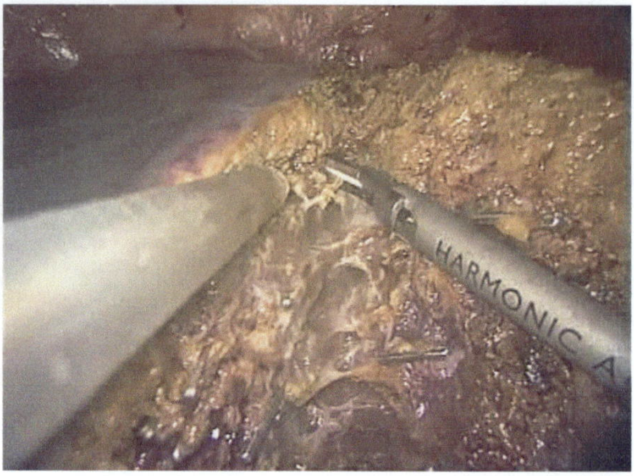

Fig. 20.3 Parenchymal transection with HARMONIC ACE® curved shears to obtain skeletonization of intrahepatic structures

tissue and small collateral braches through smaller bites of USAD and, therefore, have to be electively stapled or clipped.

When the USAD is correctly used, the cut liver surface is plain and has a brown color that helps to visualize eventual small biliary leakages, which can then be selectively secured.

Small bleedings are managed by USAD. Larger vascular and biliary structures are exposed and electively tied and cut or stapled. Once resection is complete, the liver surface must be inspected for residual bleeding or bile leakage. Biologic fibrin glue (Tissucol; Baxter, Vienna, Austria) or hemostatic gel (Floseal; Baxter, Deerfield, IL, USA) can be applied on the raw liver surface.

20.4 Complications and Results

A prospective electronic database of all patients treated by laparoscopic interventional procedures for either benign or malignant liver disease between May 2000 and December 2010 at the Department of General and Hepato-Pancreato-Biliary Surgery, S.M. Loreto Nuovo Hospital, Naples, Italy, was reviewed.

Sixty-nine procedures were carried out using USAD (UltraCision® then HARMONIC ACE®; Ethicon Endo-Surgery, Cincinnati, OH, USA), which was revealed to be a useful tool in both the dissection and parenchymal transection phases.

Blood loss, blood transfusions, need for Pringle maneuver, hospital stay, and morbidity and mortality rates were analyzed. Data are expressed as means with standard deviation. Morbidity was graded according to Clavien's classification [1].

Level of safety during transection has been satisfactory in terms of blood loss and comparable to classic technique. Among 69 liver resections, defined according to the IHPBA Brisbane 2000 classification [2], there were 21 subsegmentectomies, 18 left lateral sectionectomies, 18 segmentectomies, 5 enucleoresections, and 7 major laparoscopic resections (5 right and 2 left hepatectomies). We verified an

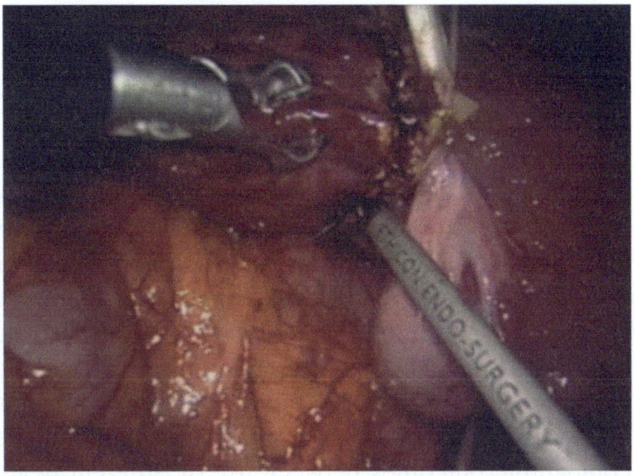

Fig. 20.4 Management of liver surface by repeated bites of HARMONIC ACE® curved shears

overall mean blood loss of 410 ml (median 400 ml, range 50–950 ml), and a median of one blood transfusion was administered in 10 % of patients. Pringle maneuver was rarely performed.

Mean hospital stay was 5.2 days (median 5 days, range 2–9 days). The overall morbidity rate was 20 %. Major morbidity occurred in two patients who respectively experienced pneumonia and acute renal failure; no postoperative biliary leakage or abscess formation was observed. Conversion rate was 6.9 %. Minor morbidity consisted of pleural effusion and transient ascites.

In the past years, risk of bleeding and concern for safe and prompt hemostasis have been the greatest reasons slowing the spread of laparoscopic approach to liver [3].

The introduction of new technological devices for efficient and fast hemostatic control during parenchymal transection greatly enhances the diffusion and safety of the laparoscopic approach in the field of liver surgery. From this perspective, new technological devices have reassured hepatic surgeons and allowed the general surgeon to approach laparoscopic liver surgery, encouraging performance of, for instance, minor liver resections for small synchronous colorectal liver metastases, instead of alternative ablative procedures.

If in open surgery technological devices can help in efficiency of procedures, in laparoscopic approach, because of limitation of spatial ranges of currently available instruments, and of the "hurdle" represented by the abdominal wall/pneumoperitoneum, they can become necessary to limit blood loss or quickly avoid unpleasant complications.

Because of its simultaneous coagulating, cutting, and sealing effect, USAD might offer many advantages over the "classic" techniques employed in open surgery.

Among the wide panorama of available devices, the USAD technology in our experience of 69 laparoscopic liver resections was revealed to be a useful tool in both the dissection and parenchymal transection phases. In fact, the Pringle maneuver was prepared but rarely applied to achieve a safe coagulating effect [4].

USAD was demonstrated to be extremely efficient in mobilizing the liver by rapid and blood-less dissection of all suspending ligaments.

When USAD is correctly used, the cut liver surface is plain and has a brown color that helps to visualize eventual small biliary leakages, which can than be selectively secured. This can explain the minimal number of typical postoperative complications, i.e., biliary leakage and local hematoma, in our series.

In recent years, we have performed laparoscopic liver resection using alternately the USAD and ultrasonic surgical aspirator system-bipolar electrocoagulator.

During use of USAD we experienced an increased sealing power of the device compared with equivalent tools available from producers in the past. Outcomes achieved by USAD increasingly allowed us to avoid employment of wet bipolar electrocoagulation or clips for vessels <5 mm in diameter, reducing operation time.

However, our experience, mainly in terms of the complication rate, revealed comparable outcomes between use of different devices.

On the other hand, we demonstrated similar outcomes in a comparative study between perioperative outcomes of open versus laparoscopic approach to liver surgery [5–10].

Our results in laparoscopic surgery can also be explained by the hemostatic effect of pneumoperitoneum, magnification of view, and minimal wall injury, provided that all required technologies are available to make procedures more efficient and safer.

References

1. Dindo D, Demartines N, Clavien PA (2004) Classification of surgical complications: a new proposal with evaluation in a cohort of 6336 patients and results of a survey. Ann Surg 240:205–213 (1. Strasberg SM)
2. Belghiti J, Clavien PA, Gadzijev E, Garden JO, Lau WY, Makuuchi M, Strong RW (2000) The Brisbane 2000 terminology of liver anatomy and resections. Terminology Committee of the International Hepato-Pancreato-Biliary Association. HPB 2:333–339
3. Cherqui D, Husson E, Hammoud R, Malassagne B, Stéphan F, Bensaid S, Rotman N, Fagniez PL (2000) Laparoscopic liver resection: a feasibility study in 30 patients. Ann Surg 232: 753–762
4. Belli G, Fantini C, D'Agostino A, Belli A, Russolillo N, Cioffi L (2005) Laparoscopic liver resection without a Pringle maneuver for HCC in cirrhotic patients. Chir Ital 57:15–25
5. Belli G, D'Agostino A, Fantini C, Cioffi L, Belli A, Limongelli P, Russo G (2009) Surgical treatment of giant liver hemangiomas by enucleation using an ultrasonically activated device (USAD). Hepatogastroenterology 56:236–239
6. Belli G, Limongelli P, Belli A, Fantini C, D'Agostino A, Cioffi L, Russo G (2008) Ultrasonically activated device for parenchymal division during open hepatectomy. HPB (Oxford) 10:234–238
7. Buell JF, Cherqui D, Geller DA, O'Rourke N, Iannitti D, Dagher I, Koffron AJ, Thomas M, Gayet B, Han HS, Wakabayashi G, Belli G, Kaneko H, Ker CG, Scatton O, Laurent A, Abdalla EK, Chaudhury P, Dutson E, Gamblin C, D'Angelica M, Nagorney D, Testa G, Labow D, Manas D, Poon RT, Nelson H, Martin R, Clary B, Pinson WC, Martinie J, Vauthey JN, Goldstein R, Roayaie S, Barlet D, Espat J, Abecassis M, Rees M, Fong Y, McMasters KM, Broelsch C, Busuttil R, Belghiti J, Strasberg S (2009) World Consensus Conference on Laparoscopic Surgery.

The international position on laparoscopic liver surgery: The Louisville Statement, 2008. Ann Surg 250:825–830
8. Belli G, Limongelli P, Fantini C, D'Agostino A, Cioffi L, Belli A, Russo G (2009) Laparoscopic and open treatment of hepatocellular carcinoma in patients with cirrhosis. Br J Surg 96:1041–1048
9. Dagher I, Belli G, Fantini C, Laurent A, Tayar C, Lainas P, Tranchart H, Franco D, Cherqui D (2010) Laparoscopic hepatectomy for hepatocellular carcinoma: a European experience. J Am Coll Surg 211:16–23
10. Belli G, Fantini C, D'Agostino A, Cioffi L, Langella S, Russolillo N, Belli A (2007) Laparoscopic versus open liver resection for hepatocellular carcinoma in patients with histologically proven cirrhosis: short- and middle-term results. Surg Endosc 21:2004–2011

Laparoscopic Hepatic Transection Using Bipolar Radiofrequency Ablation (EnSeal)

21

Keith M. Baldwin, Ponnandai Somasundar, Steven C. Katz and N. Joseph Espat

21.1 Introduction

Currently, on a global basis, an increasing number of hepatic resections are being performed for benign and malignant hepatic tumors. Simultaneously, populations continue to increase in age and number of medical comorbidities. For those requiring hepatic resection, modalities such as laparoscopy will prove to be valuable adjuncts.

Inherent technical challenges in laparoscopic hepatic surgery, such as management of large bile ducts and hepatic blood vessels, have been addressed by routine use of articulating endomechanical stapling devices. However, hepatic

---

Electronic Supplementary Material The online version of this article (doi:10.1007/978-88-470-2622-3_21) contains supplementary material which is available to authorized users.

Contribution from the Department of Surgery, Roger Williams Medical Center, Providence, RI.

K. M. Baldwin · P. Somasundar · S. C. Katz · N. Joseph Espat (✉)
Department of Surgery, Roger Williams Medical Center, 825 Chalkstone Avenue, Providence, RI 02908, USA
e-mail: jespat@hepaticsurgery.com

K. M. Baldwin
e-mail: kbaldwin@chartercare.org

P. Somasundar
e-mail: psomasundar@chartercare.org

S. C. Katz
e-mail: skatz@chartercare.org

I. Di Carlo (ed.), *Open, Laparoscopic and Robotic Hepatic Transection*,
DOI: 10.1007/978-88-470-2622-3_21,

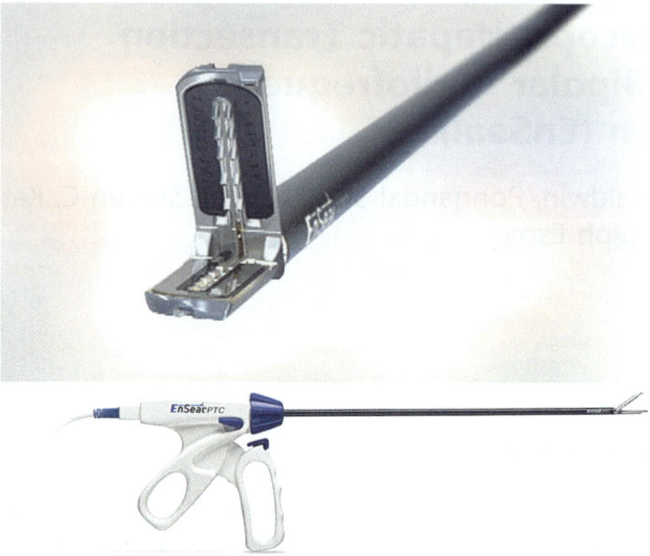

Fig. 21.1 Design and ergonomics of the BRFA device. Simultaneous vessel sealing and cutting can be performed. Jaw size is comparable to the ultrasonic shears or 5-mm LigaSure device, and it rotates 360° (image courtesy of Ethicon Endo-Surgery, Inc.)

parenchymal transection under laparoscopic conditions remains a significant challenge without a defined optimal technique.

Traditional crush-clamp techniques utilizing clips and suture ligation remain either technically unfeasible or too laborious for the laparoscopic approach. As such, various energy-based (thermal generating) devices have been introduced which are able to simultaneously seal, coagulate, and cut hepatic parenchyma and associated small vessels (<7 mm).

Precoagulation transection (PCT) refers to the use of such energy devices, and usually relies on thermal energy in the form of monopolar, ultrasonic or bipolar delivery [1]. Protein denaturing and resultant vessel and bile duct fusion translate into more controlled operative bleeding and potentially lower rates of biliary leakage [2].

21.2 Device Description and Use in Laparoscopy

At present, the authors' preferred energy device for laparoscopic hepatic parenchymal PCT is the bipolar radiofrequency device (BRF, EnSeal; Ethicon Endo-Surgery, Cincinnati OH). The device allows the surgeon to seal and transect small to large vessels and tissue bundles, and is approved for transection of blood vessels up to 7 mm in size (Fig. 21.1) [3]. In a comparison of four energy-based vascular sealing/cutting instruments in porcine arteries, the seal formed by this BRF device

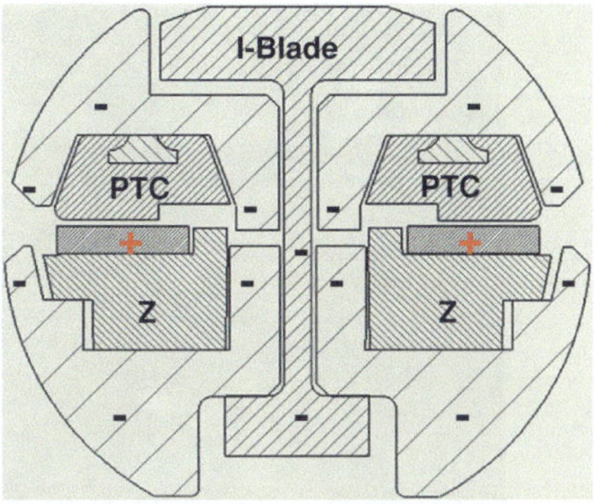

Fig. 21.2 Cross-sectional view of the closed BRFA jaw. Positive electrodes are buried within the jaw so that the flow of energy occurs inward, minimizing thermal spread outside the jaw. I = I-blade; PTC = conductive nanoparticles; (+) = positive electrode; (−) = negative electrode (image courtesy of Ethicon Endo-Surgery, Inc.)

was found to tolerate the highest burst pressure at seven times normal systolic pressure [4].

Bipolar RF energy is delivered using the "line-of-sight" principle where energy is only transferred between the electrodes of the upper and lower jaw. The jaws of the bipolar RFA act as two negative electrodes, and the positive electrode is embedded in the inner portion of the lower jaw; thus, the flow of energy is inward (Fig. 21.2). Additionally, a polymer with conductive particles is embedded in the upper jaw. It employs a novel nanotechnology to control the heat delivered to the jaws. At about 100 °C the conductive particles reach significant molecular distance so as to stop conduction of energy in that part of the jaw, while another part of the jaw may continue heating (Fig. 21.3). As a result, the lateral thermal spread of the device is 1 mm or less, as compared with 1.93 mm and 2.11 mm, respectively, for the ultrasonic shears and bipolar vessel sealer (LigaSure) in one animal study [5].

The BRF device is available in 25 cm and 35 cm shaft lengths, and the circumference is amenable for use through a 5-mm port. The BRF can be used for either laparoscopic or laparotomy-based procedures. Its laparoscopic use is described herein. The BRF jaw is blunt and is available in either a straight or slightly curved configuration, depending on surgeon preference. The presence and use of a blade lock-out flip switch (toggle) also enable the device to function as a blunt dissector and grasper .

Unlike other energy devices, sealing and cutting occur in one surgeon-controlled movement which may be performed slowly or quickly depending on the thickness of the tissue being divided during PCT. As the device heats, the cutting I-beam blade can be deployed at any time and at any speed as desired by the operating surgeon. After the blade reaches the tip of the jaw, the generator audibly indicates that maximum tissue impedance has been achieved, thus notifying the surgeon that the jaw can be released. There is a toggle switch that changes the device from sealing and cutting mode to sealing-only mode. In this mode the blade will not advance, making it safe for grasping and for hemostasis where cutting is not desired.

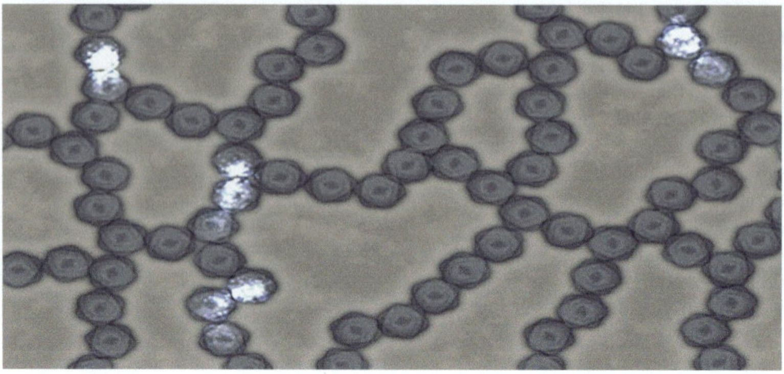

Fig. 21.3 Nanoparticles embedded within the jaw of the device cease conducting when temperature reaches 100 °C, however the effect is regional and other areas within the jaw may continue heating if the temperature is <100 °C (image courtesy of Ethicon Endo-Surgery, Inc.)

21.3 Technique Description

Principles of this BRF hepatic laparoscopic PCT technique include many which are common to laparoscopic hepatic surgery in general. Low central venous pressure (CVP) anesthesia is utilized to maintain pretransection CVP <5 mmHg. The hepatic lesion is identified with use of intraoperative ultrasound (IOUS) in all but the most peripheral lesions. Five-millimeter trocars are used in a typical upper gastrointestinal (GI) laparoscopy configuration, except for one or two 12-mm trocars which facilitate the use of IOUS and eventual introduction of endomechanical staplers for larger vessels. Formal inflow occlusion (Pringle) is not routinely used, and steep reverse Trendelenburg position is employed both to allow gravity retraction of viscera and to reduce CVP.

Hepatic transection proceeds as follows: monopolar electrocautery is used with intraoperative ultrasound to score Glisson's capsule as a guide to ensure appropriate margins. Parenchymal transection begins by introduction of the BRF device into the scored parenchyma. The jaws of the device are gently closed to compress the tissue but without crushing. PCT begins with activation of the trigger, and deployment of the cutting blade may begin, slowly for thicker tissue and more rapidly for thin layers. PCT of approximately 1 cm, from activation to the generator signal that impedance has been reached and cutting is complete, takes between 3 and 10 s depending on tissue thickness.

The plane of transection is then continued by keeping the device in the same orientation and simply advancing along the scored cautery line, without removing the instrument jaw from the tissue. Importantly, the jaw should be kept at the same level of depth and advanced gradually to obtain a consistent PCT plane. The process is repeated throughout the anterior and posterior surfaces of the liver, following the scored line. Once the more superficial layers are exposed, the process is repeated on deeper layers for 2–3 cm of depth, or until larger hepatic veins or ducts are identified. Endomechanical staplers are used to divide these structures.

Important caveats to the use of the BRF device are as follows: The BRF will not activate in the presence of a metal staple, and the generator will alarm. In these cases, cautery or scissors should be used to gently transect a few millimeters beyond the area of the staples before the BRF is used again. Also, if very thick tissues are transected, the I-blade of the device may "jump," resulting in tissue transaction without coagulation. This can be avoided by taking thinner tissue bites with the jaw and closing the handle in a slow, controlled manner.

Although the device is approved for blood vessels up to 7 mm in size, surgeon judgment should be used when deciding whether the BRF or endomechanical staplers are appropriate for hemostasis. Particular caution should be used when caudate lobe vessels are divided [6]. Actual clinical data testing the device in vivo largely stem from colorectal surgery applications and its use in laparoscopic nephrectomy [7–9]. In a series of 71 laparoscopic colectomies, a total of 224 named vessels (including 42 inferior mesenteric arteries and 45 inferior mesenteric veins) were divided with the bipolar RFA alone with a single-application seal rate of 98.7 %. Three large vessels required a clip, and there was no postoperative bleeding [9].

Although controlled data utilizing energy devices for laparoscopic hepatic transection are scarce, the authors' initial experience with the BRF has been positive. In the previously published series of 18 laparoscopic resections utilizing the BRF (2 hemihepatectomies, 4 left lateral segmentectomies, 3 right posterior sectorectomies, and 9 atypical resections), estimated blood loss was 178 ± 53 ml, including concomitant colectomies and other procedures. Mean operative time was 114 ± 56 min for the liver resections. A purely laparoscopic technique was used in most cases, utilizing hand-assisted methods only in more complicated cases [10, 11]. As with any laparoscopic technique, there is a learning curve with the use of the BRF, mainly relating to the concomitant heating and cutting motions, which differs from some energy devices currently in use. The authors' general observation is that within 2–3 cases most trainees are comfortable with the device. Clearly, surgeon comfort with a particular device and technique plays a large role in the success of any complex laparoscopic procedure.

References

1. Lupo L, Gallerani A, Panzera P et al. (2007) Randomized clinical trial of radiofrequency-assisted versus clamp-crushing liver resection. Br J Surg 94:278–291
2. Sahin DA, Kusaslan R, Sahin O et al. (2007) Histopathological effects of bipolar vessel sealing devices on liver parenchyma and comparison with suture method: an experimental study. Eur Surg Res 39:111–117
3. EnSeal product information, Ethicon Endo-Surgery, Cincinnati, OH

4. Person B, Vivas DA, Ruiz D et al. (2008) Comparison of four energy-based vascular sealing and cutting instruments: a porcine model. Surg Endosc 22:534–538
5. Golstein SL, Harold KL, Lentzner A et al. (2002) Comparison of thermal spread after ureteral ligation with the laparo-sonic ultrasonic shears and the Ligasure system. J Laparoendosc Adv Surg Tech 12:61–63
6. Helton S, Van Cott C, Zuckerman R (2009). Enseal bipolar cutting device enables safe and bloodless hepatic subsegmentectomy. Presented at the IHPBA 8th European Congress, June 2009
7. Smaldone MC, Gibbons EP, Jackman SV (2008) Laparoscopic nephrectomy using the Enseal tissue sealing and haemostasis system; successful therapeutic application of nanotechnology. JSLS 12:213–216
8. Albert M, Atallah S, Larach S, Parra-Davila E (2009) Vessel sealing in laparoscopic colonic surgery. Presented at: 2009 scientific session of the society of American gastrointestinal and endoscopic surgeons (SAGES), Phoenix, AZ, 22–25 April 2009
9. Quinteros F, Maricek S, Clinton J, et al. (2009) Experience with EnSeal vessel-sealing device in colectomy. Presented at the 2009 scientific session of the society of American gastrointestinal and endoscopic surgeons (SAGES), Phoenix, AZ, 22–25 April 2009
10. Somasundar P, Boutros C, Helton WS, Espat NJ (2009) Evaluation of a bipolar radiofrequency device for laparoscopic hepatic transaction: technique and clinical experience in 18 patients. HPB 11:145–149
11. Alemi F, Kwon E, Chiu J, Aoki H, Stewart L, Corvera CU (2011) Laparoscopic treatment of liver tumors using a two-needle probe bipolar radiofrequency ablation device. HPB (Oxford) 13(9):656–64

Part III
Robotic Transection

Robotic Liver Resection

22

Ki-Hun Kim and Gi-Hong Choi

22.1 Introduction

Minimally invasive surgical procedures have gained widespread acceptance among surgeons and patients. Sophisticated technologies, such as digital optics, energized dissection systems, and medical instrumentation, enable surgeons to perform a number of complex operations laparoscopically, including organ procurement from live donors, in which the safety of healthy volunteers cannot be compromised. These advanced minimally invasive procedures require surgeons to have highly developed laparoscopic skills, including suturing, knot-tying, and complex bimanual manipulation. However, conventional laparoscopic surgery has limitations, including reduced freedom of movement within the abdominal cavity and the fact that it provides two-dimensional views of a three-dimensional operative field. Recently, the da Vinci surgical system (Intuitive Surgical, Inc., Sunnyvale, CA, USA), a robotic surgical system, was approved by the US Food and

Electronic Supplementary Material The online version of this article (doi:10.1007/978-88-470-2622-3_22) contains supplementary material which is available to authorized users.

K.-H. Kim (✉)
Division of Hepatobiliary Surgery and Liver Transplantation, Department of Surgery, Ulsan University, Asan Medical Center, 388-1 Pungnap-dong, Songpa-gu, Seoul 138-736, Republic of Korea
e-mail: khkim620@amc.seoul.kr

G.-H. Choi
Department of Surgery, Yonsei University Health System, 250 Seongsanno, Seodaemoon-gu, Seoul 120-752, Republic of Korea
e-mail: Choigh@yuhs.ac

I. Di Carlo (ed.), *Open, Laparoscopic and Robotic Hepatic Transection*, DOI: 10.1007/978-88-470-2622-3_22, © Springer-Verlag Italia 2012

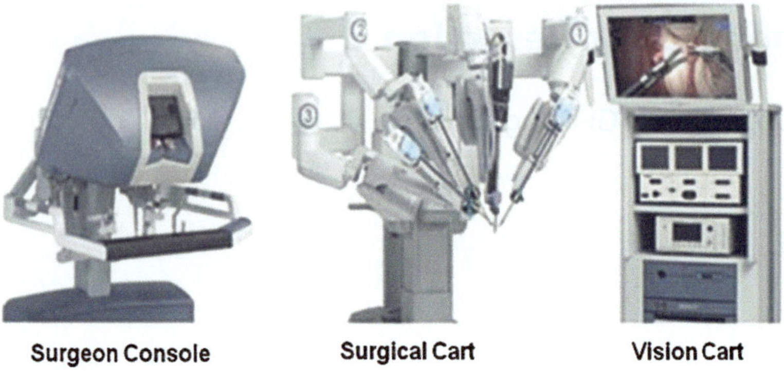

Fig. 22.1 da Vinci surgical system

Drug Administration for use in surgery. The da Vinci system is the only commercially available therapeutic robotic system on the market and allows surgeons to perform advanced laparoscopic procedures with greater ease. Similar to a human hand, the robotic articulating instruments translate the natural movements of the surgeon's hand into precise movements inside the abdominal cavity. The system allows three-dimensional views of the operative field, has tremor filtration capacity, and permits seven degrees of freedom. This allows surgeons to dexterously perform delicate dissections and precise intracorporeal suturing. The significant advantages of robotic surgery have expanded the scope of surgical procedures that can be performed through minimally invasive techniques. This chapter describes the operative procedure of robotic liver resection.

22.2 Device Description

22.2.1 da Vinci Surgical System

The da Vinci surgical system consists of three parts, including surgical cart, vision cart, and surgeon console (Fig. 22.1). The surgical cart is composed of four robotic arms, being connected to the surgeon console via a cable. The center arm holds the camera system, and the three lateral arms hold the surgical instruments. The multiple robotic arm and distal instrument joints allow seven degrees of freedom, as the human wrist in open surgery. There are two camera control units in the vision cart. Two image synchronizers and a focus controller provide the surgeon sitting at the console with a high-quality three-dimensional view of the surgical field with adjustable magnification. The surgeon console consists of the binocular viewer of the Insite vision system, the instrument controllers, a series of foot control pedals, and the computer hardware and software. The surgeon sits at the console with elbows resting on a padded bar.

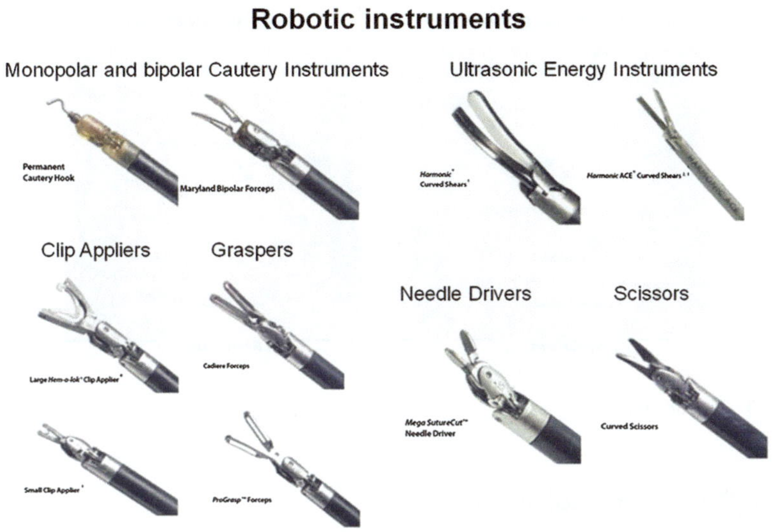

Fig. 22.2 Robotic instruments

An ergonomic operating position is established by adjusting the height of the chair and the position of the foot pedals and maintained by using the clutch pedal to reposition the surgeon's arms and hands during surgery. Another advantage of the da Vinci surgical system is that the digitization of the surgeon's hand movements on the controls allows elimination of surgeon tremor and production of motion scaling (up to five times).

22.2.2 Instruments

The instruments currently available in robotic liver resection are shown in Fig. 22.2. A monopolar cautery hook and Maryland bipolar forceps are mainly used to dissect the hilar structures and ligaments around the liver. Major vessels such as hepatic artery and portal vein are ligated using robotic clip applier. Three sizes of clip appliers with small titanium clip, Hem-o-lok medium-large, and large polymer clips are available according to vessel size. A needle driver can be used for suture ligation of either portal vein branches to the caudate lobe during mobilization of the right portal vein or injured vessels. Harmonic scalpel and Maryland bipolar forceps are mainly used to transect liver parenchyma. Maryland bipolar forceps is also used to control minor bleeding at the cut surface of the liver and finely dissect intraparenchymal major hepatic vein branches during parenchymal transection. The Cadière forceps is usually mounted on the third robotic arm and used for retraction and exposure.

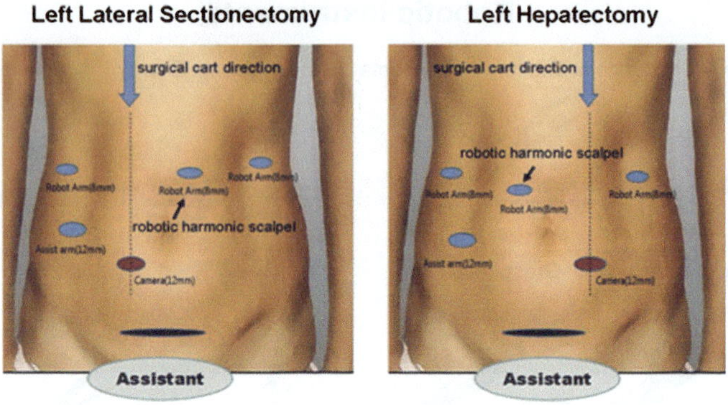

Fig. 22.3 Trocar position

22.2.3 Operative Indications

The indications for robotic liver resection are similar to those for laparoscopic liver resection as mentioned in the 2008 Louisville Statement. There was a consensus that laparoscopic liver surgery should be limited to selected patients. The best candidates for laparoscopic liver resection are patients with solitary lesions that are located in the peripheral liver segments (segments II–VI) and are 5 cm or less in diameter. Most types of liver resection can be performed laparoscopically, including major liver resections (i.e., right or left hepatectomies). However, such extensive resections should be performed only by experienced surgeons who are already competent at performing more limited laparoscopic resections.

22.3 Technique Description

22.3.1 Robotic Left Hepatectomy

The patient is placed supine in 15° reverse Trendelenburg position, with an assistant standing between the patient's legs. A 12-mm trocar for the robotic camera is placed either below or above the left side of the patient's umbilicus. Carbon dioxide is insufflated, and pneumoperitoneum is maintained at 12 mmHg. Three 8-mm trocars are placed in the right subcostal, paramedian, and left subcostal areas. A 12-mm trocar for an assistant is placed in the right lower quadrant area. The surgical cart of the four-arm da Vinci surgical system is placed and docked coming from the patient's head toward the camera port, and the trocar for the robotic harmonic scalpel is placed along the target lesion (Fig. 22.3). The surgeon moves to the surgeon's cart to control the robotic arms. The assistant stands between the patient's legs to change robotic instruments and perform clipping, stapling, suction, irrigation, and retraction through a 12-mm trocar placed

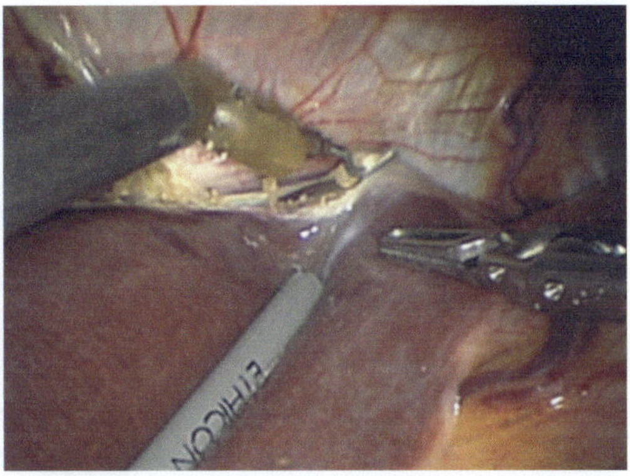

Fig. 22.4 Left liver mobilization

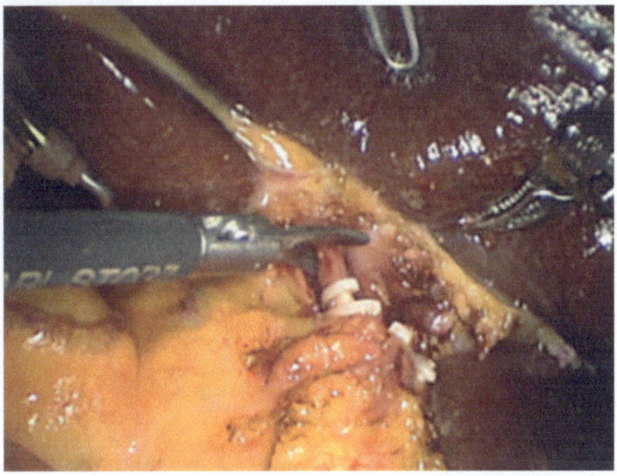

Fig. 22.5 Cutting the left hepatic artery

at the right lower quadrant. The right subcostal port is used for liver retraction with the robotic arm. The left triangular and falciform ligaments are divided with the permanent cautery hook for full left liver mobilization (Fig. 22.4). Using a Maryland bipolar forceps, the left hepatic artery and portal vein are dissected and identified. These vessels may be divided using metal or Hem-o-lok® clips (Weck Closure System, Research Triangle Park, NC, USA) or can be ligated with the robotic needle holder (Figs. 22.5, 22.6). Parenchymal division is carried out along the demarcation line using the robotic harmonic scalpel (Fig. 22.7). The larger Glissonian pedicles are ligated, clipped, and divided. No Pringle maneuver is used during parenchymal division. The left hepatic duct and left hepatic vein are exposed after complete division of the remnant hepatic parenchyma and are divided using an Endo-GIA stapler (Covidien, Mansfield, MA, USA) (Fig. 22.8). The specimen is placed in an endobag inserted through a 12-mm trocar and retrieved through a 10-cm suprapubic incision site. A closed suction drain is inserted to prevent fluid collection, and fibrin glue is applied to the resection site after hemostasis and biliostasis have been achieved (Fig. 22.9).

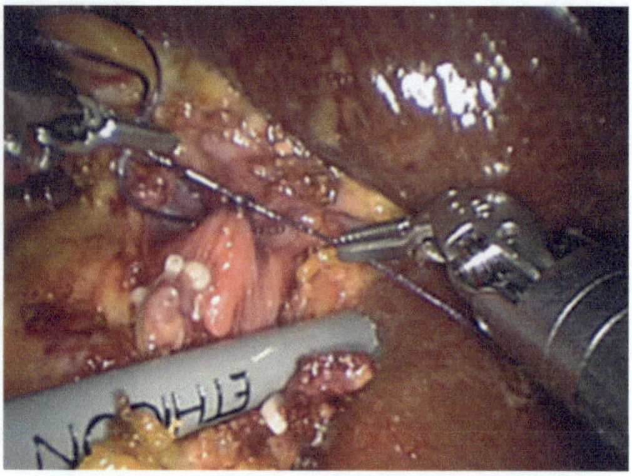

Fig. 22.6 Ligation of the left portal vein

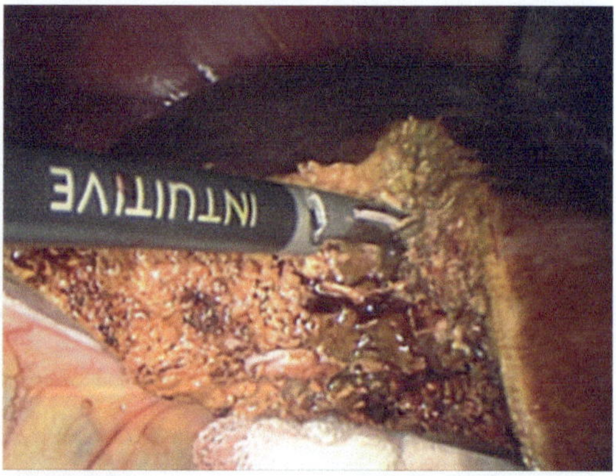

Fig. 22.7 Division of the hepatic parenchyma

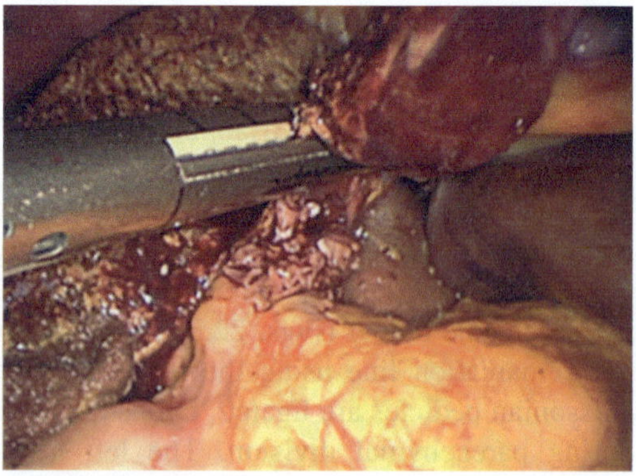

Fig. 22.8 Division of the left hepatic duct using Endo-GIA

22.3.2 Robotic Left Lateral Sectionectomy

A 12-mm trocar for the robotic camera is placed below or above the right side of the patient's umbilicus. The trocar for the robotic harmonic scalpel is placed on the left side of the patient along the target lesion (Fig. 22.3). The left lateral section is

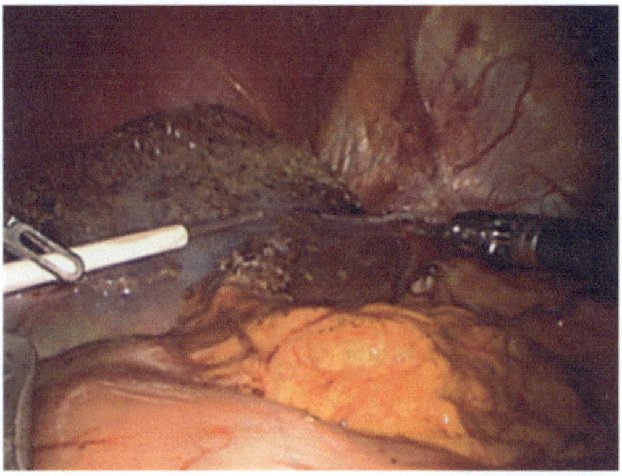

Fig. 22.9 Application of fibrin glue

mobilized, as is the case during the left hepatectomy. The left subcostal port is used for liver retraction by the robotic arm. The Glissonian pedicles of segment II and III are divided using an Endo-GIA stapler or individual ligation. The left hepatic vein is exposed after complete transection of the hepatic parenchyma and is divided using an Endo-GIA stapler. The procedures for specimen retrieval, closed suction drain insertion, and fibrin glue application are similar to left hepatectomy.

22.3.3 Robotic Right Hepatectomy

Five ports are used. The 12-mm camera port is placed in the right periumbilical area. The first and second robotic arm ports are placed in the left and right upper quadrant areas, respectively. The third robotic arm port is placed near the left anterior axillary line and is usually used for exposure and retraction. The assistant's port is placed at the umbilicus. This placement can provide good access for clipping, suction, and vascular stapling during parenchymal transection (Fig. 22.10). After induction of pneumoperitoneum, the robotic arm ports and the assistant's port are placed. The patient is positioned in 15° reverse Trendelenburg position, and the surgical cart is installed. The round ligament and falciform ligament are sectioned with the robotic harmonic scalpel mounted on the first robotic arm. When the dissection approaches the bare area, the permanent cautery hook can be used to dissect the coronary ligament. The dissection of the anterior half of the coronary ligament proceeds until the anterior side of the inferior vena cava (IVC) and the right hepatic vein are exposed. For mobilization of the right lobe of the liver, the third-arm lifting method has been introduced by Guilianotti et al. The Cadière forceps, mounted on the third robotic arm, is used to retract the right lobe of the liver upward, exposing the hepatorenal ligament and the right triangular ligament. The dissection is conducted with the permanent cautery hook and the Maryland bipolar forceps. The dissection of the right side of the IVC starts at the caudate process of the caudate lobe. The short hepatic veins and the vena cava ligament are dissected and ligated with Hem-o-lok® clips (Fig. 22.11). The

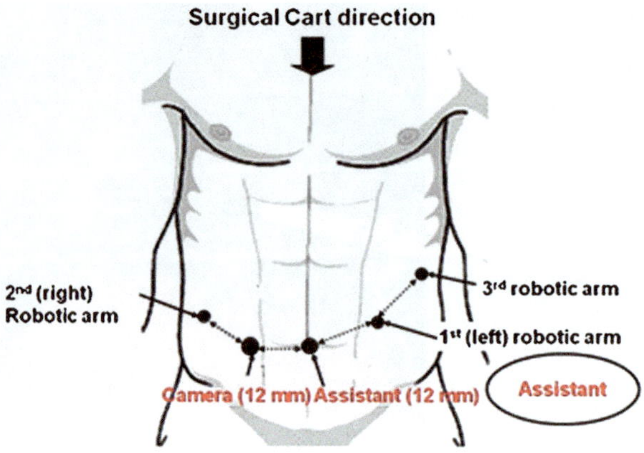

Fig. 22.10 Port placement for right hepatectomy

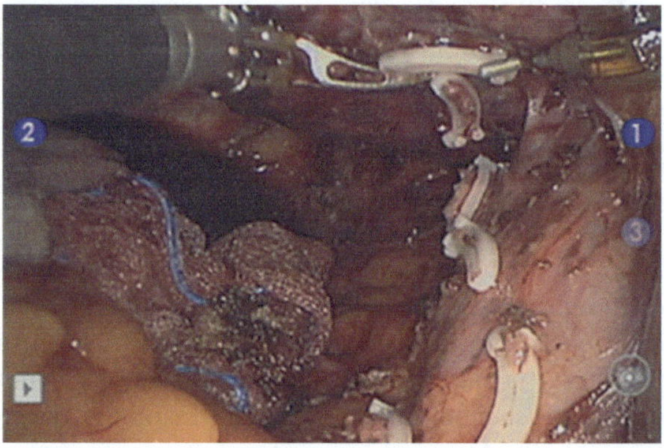

Fig. 22.11 Mobilization of the right liver and dissection of IVC

hilum is exposed by retracting either the inferior surface of the liver or the gallbladder with the third robotic arm. The right hepatic artery is identified at the right side of the common bile duct and is sectioned after applying Hem-o-lok® clips (Fig. 22.12). The right portal vein usually has one or two small branches to the caudate lobe, which should be divided after proximal transfixing stitches are placed (Fig. 22.13). The right portal vein is completely mobilized and then divided between the Hem-o-lok clips (Fig. 22.14). The parenchymal transection is conducted following the ischemic demarcation line using the harmonic curved shears and the Maryland bipolar forceps. To expose the parenchymal transection plane, Giulianotti et al. applied stay stitches at the resection margins, and used the third robotic arm for retraction and exposure. The authors developed a rubber band retraction method. Two rubber bands are fixed at the right and left resection margins using stay stitches. The other end of the rubber band is pulled out and

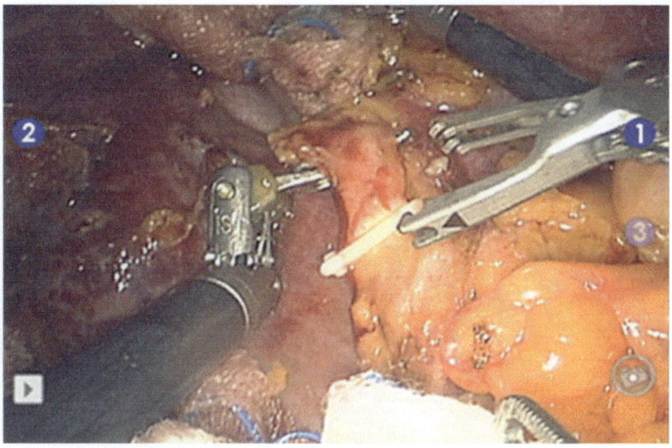

Fig. 22.12 Ligation of the right hepatic artery

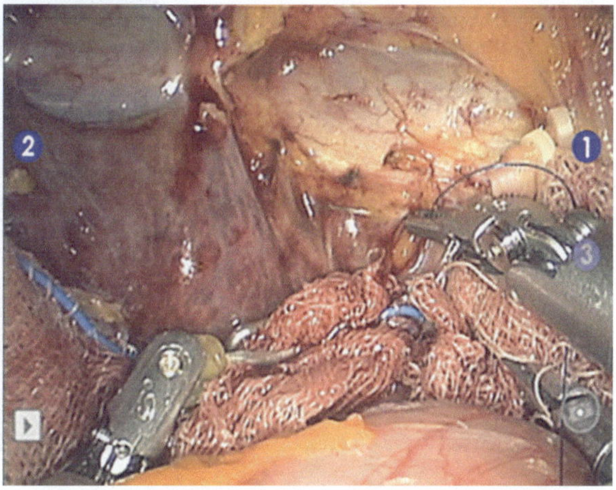

Fig. 22.13 Transfixing stitches of the portal vein branch

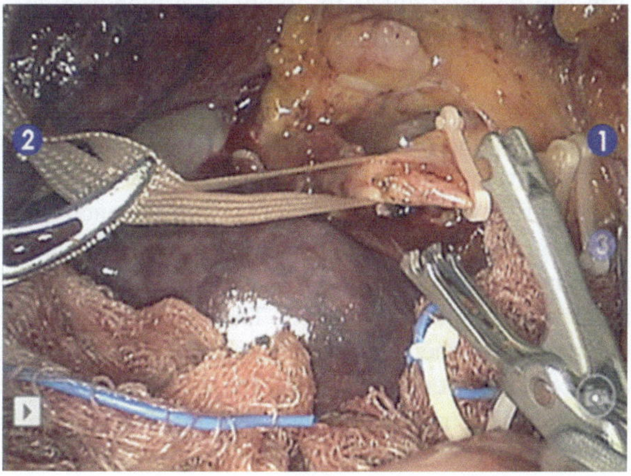

Fig. 22.14 Ligation of the right portal vein

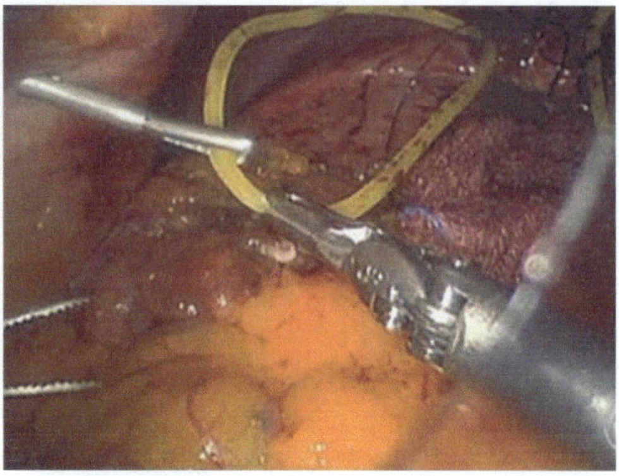

Fig. 22.15 Fixation of two rubber bands for liver retraction

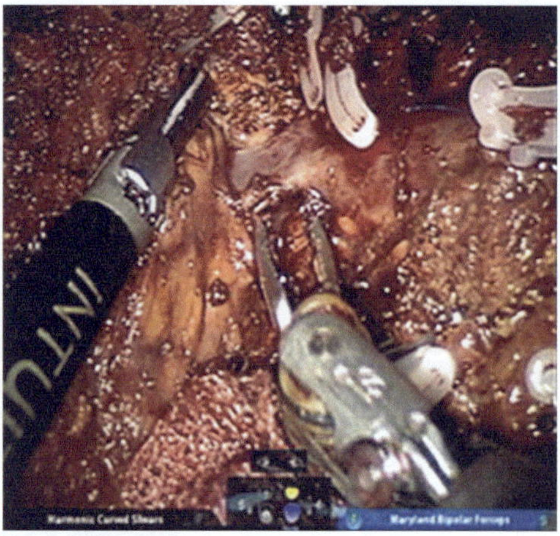

Fig. 22.16 Dissection of segment VIII branch of MHV

fixed with appropriate tension at the outside operative field (Fig. 22.15). The rubber band provides a stable parenchymal transection plane, and the third robotic arm can be used either to compress a bleeding site or to retract the liver during parenchymal transection. Bleeding from the small Glissonian pedicles can be well controlled by the robotic harmonic scalpel. In the deep liver parenchyma, major middle hepatic vein branches, such as segment V and segment VIII, are carefully dissected and divided (Fig. 22.16). The liver parenchyma around the hilar plate is carefully removed, and then the right bile duct, including the hilar plate, is sectioned after ligation (Fig. 22.17). The parenchyma is gradually dissected in the direction of the right hepatic vein. Finally, the right hepatic vein is identified and is sectioned using an Endo-GIA stapler (Fig. 22.18). The remaining coronary ligament is completely dissected. The specimen is placed in a large plastic bag. The cut surface of the liver is irrigated, and fine bleeding is controlled. Fibrin glue is applied to the cut surface of the liver. The surgical cart is unlocked, and the specimen is retrieved through a 10-cm Pfannenstiel incision.

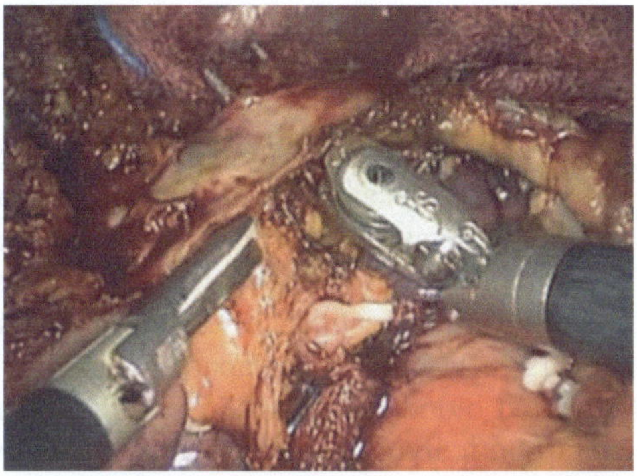

Fig. 22.17 Dissection of the right bile duct

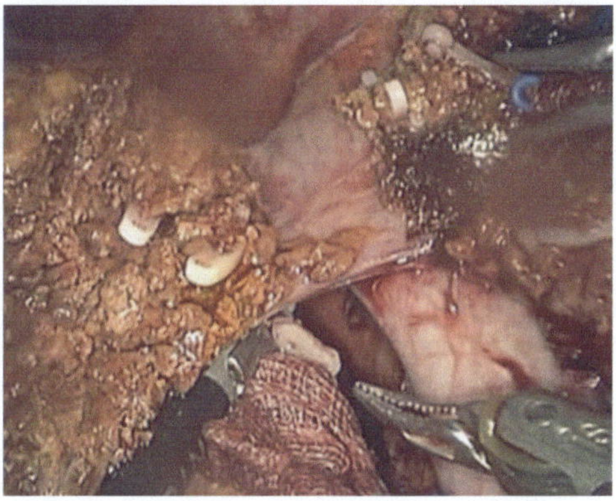

Fig. 22.18 Dissection and complete exposure of RHV

22.4 Complications and Results

Thirteen robotic liver resections (10 left lateral sectionectomy and 3 left hepatectomy) and 17 laparoscopic liver resections (11 left hepatectomy and 6 left lateral sectionectomy) were compared. There was no significant difference in mean operative time (robotic versus laparoscopic, 291.5 ± 85.1 versus 240.9 ± 68.6 min; $p = 0.082$) or mean estimated blood loss (robotic versus laparoscopic, 388.5 ± 65.0 versus 342.6 ± 84.7 ml; $p = 0.114$) between the two groups. There was no complication in the robotic liver resection group. The only different item, mean medical cost, was higher in the robotic liver resection group (robotic versus laparoscopic: 11,475 ± 2,174 versus 6,762 ± 1,436 USD; $p = 0.001$).

Right hepatectomy was performed in six patients. There were six hepatocellular carcinomas and one intrahepatic duct stones. One patient underwent colon resection simultaneously. The average operation time and estimated blood loss were 724 min (range 648–812 min) and 629 ml (range 100–1,500 ml), respectively. Two patients received perioperative transfusion. There was one conversion to open surgery due to severe hilar adhesion and anatomic deformation in patient with intrahepatic duct stone during hilum dissection. There were three complications, including one intra-abdominal fluid collection (grade I), one superficial wound infection (grade IIIa), and colon anastomotic leakage (grade IIIb). Mean length of hospital stay was 11.7 days (range 9–46 days).

Robotic surgical systems offer an alternative to laparoscopic liver resection for minimally invasive liver resections. Well-trained surgeons can perform both major and minor liver resections through the robotic approach. Although little data regarding robotic liver resection have been reported, robotic liver resection appears to be similar to laparoscopic liver resection in terms of operative time, estimated blood loss, hospital stay, and time to resumption of normal diet. However, robotic liver resection is more expensive than laparoscopic resection. Robotic liver resection may become more popular for minimally invasive liver surgery if upgraded robotic surgical systems can be developed that are smaller, cost less, have good tactile feedback, and incorporate various hepatic parenchymal transection tools such as CUSA and LigaSure.

References

Idrees K, Bartlett DL (2010) Robotic liver surgery. Surg Clin North Am 90:761–774

Giulianotti PC, Coratti A, Sbrana F, et al. (2011a) Robotic liver surgery: results for 70 resection. Surgery 149:29–39

Choi SB, Park JS, Kim JK, et al. (2008) Early experiences of robotic-assisted laparoscopic liver resection. Yonsei Med J 49:632–638

Buell JF, Cherqui D, Geller DA, et al. (2008) The international position on laparoscopic liver surgery: the Louisville statement. Ann Surg 250:825–830

Kim KH, Jung DH, Park KM, et al. (2011) Comparison of open and laparoscopic live donor left lateral sectionectomy. Br J Surg 98:1302–1308

Giulianotti PC, Sbrana F, Coratti A, et al. (2011b) Totally robotic right hepatectomy: surgical technique and outcomes. Arch Surg 146:844–850

Index

I. Di Carlo (ed.), *Open, Laparoscopic and Robotic Hepatic Transection,*
DOI: 10.1007/978-88-470-2622-3,

GPSR Compliance

The European Union's (EU) General Product Safety Regulation (GPSR) is a set of rules that requires consumer products to be safe and our obligations to ensure this.

If you have any concerns about our products, you can contact us on ProductSafety@springernature.com

In case Publisher is established outside the EU, the EU authorized representative is:

Springer Nature Customer Service Center GmbH
Europaplatz 3
69115 Heidelberg, Germany

Batch number: 10772487

Printed by Printforce, the Netherlands